THE
SILENT
BATTLE

E MAN'S FIGHT FOR FREEDOM

RICH MOORE

THE SILENT BATTLE

One Man's Fight for Freedom

© Copyright 2011 & 2016 by Rich Moore

Printed in the United States of America
ALL RIGHTS RESERVED
www.puredesire.org

Published by

Pure Desire Ministries International
www.puredesire.org | Gresham, Oregon | May 2016
First Edition, 2011

ISBN 978-1-943291-81-6

TABLE OF CONTENTS

DEDICATION

THIS BOOK IS DEDICATED TO THOSE WHO HAVE WALKED WITH ME OVER THE YEARS

First, I would like to thank the Lord for saving my life and bringing peace back into it. There were so many times I wanted to run, but God never let me go. He believed in me when I felt no one else did.

I would like to thank my wife, Deneen, who has shown me what strength looks like. I love her dedication to the Lord. She has continued to support me and believes that I can overcome my past. She truly is a blessing in my life—someone I will cherish always.

To my two beautiful children, Christian and Courtney, who have inspired me to be a better father: Thank you for your love.

To my family for their support, love and forgiveness: I never thought we could overcome so much pain and loss, but through this, God has blessed us all. Thanks, Mom, for never giving up on me and praying for me every day. You were always the one constant in my life. To Mark, my dad, thank you for walking through the healing journey with me, which I know wasn't easy; thanks for being the dad you didn't have to be.

Dr. Ted Roberts. What can I say, Ted? You have truly been an inspiration to me. Thank you for being so transparent during your teachings and for sharing the darkest times of your life. I soaked up every word, thinking if you could make it through your stuff, I could also make it through mine. Thank you for developing Pure Desire. God knew the tools I needed, and it was birthed out of you. I don't think I can articulate the words to express what you have done for me. I am truly grateful.

Harry Flanagan. Thank you for being there and investing in me. I have learned much from your teachings and truly appreciate the friendship we have. You, right along with Dr. Ted, have helped steer me in the direction I needed to go; you kept loving me when I did not love myself.

Mike Townsend. Thanks for showing me that I was loved during such a tough time, for being the first friend I shared my story with in that pizza place so many years back. Thank you, Mike, for being there for me.

And to my brother Pat: If ever I wanted to be like someone growing up, it was you. The word "hero" has so many meanings, but you are a hero to me; you have shown me so much grace and forgiveness that I cannot even comprehend. Through those very tough years, and even today, I see you as a rock—solid in your faith, family, and career. I will always look up to you. I saw God in a new light through you. I am blessed to call you my brother. Thank you for giving me a second chance—and for not giving up on me.

Sugar Carpenter. Thank you for not letting me say "fine" when you asked me how I was doing. You always made me communicate at deeper levels.

Dave and Nancy McMillan, Gil And Rosemary Albelo. Thanks for being there for me, praying for me and never giving up. Thank you for the prayer covering you provided for our family.

There are so many more people I could list. Thank you to all who have walked with me. You are all truly remarkable men and women. I thank God for placing you all in my life.

BY DR. TED ROBERTS

I immediately liked Rich the first time I met him. He has a heart that profoundly impresses you. Most folks are probably impressed with his physical size, but I was taken aback by the enormity of his heart. Yet, at the same time, I could sense an avalanche of pain within. This book is about the incredible miracles the Holy Spirit has done in his life to heal that pain.

If you have ever struggled with sexual issues in your life, this book will give you hope! If you have a friend who is wrestling with the hellish hooks of sexual bondage, this book is a *must* read; it will give you some very practical tools to help him find healing.

You may not be battling with sexual difficulties, but if you have ever struggled with anger and forgiveness—once again, this book is for you!

It is more than a personal testimony; it looks deeply at a man's soul in the anguishing and messy process of becoming who God has called him to be. Therefore, in a sense, it is a graphic portrayal of all of us.

Rich reminds me of a dear friend I had in military flight training. Like Rich, he came in the extra large size; he was enormous for a fighter pilot. We both flew out to the aircraft carrier to be qualified in a single seat fighter. He was positioned ahead of me on the catapult for our first shot. The jet blast deflector rose up, blocking my view as my friend came to full power prior to launch. I felt the explosion of the catapult fling him off the front end as the carrier plowed relentlessly through the slate blue sea. Once my view of the bow was clear, I gasped! My friend was fighting for his life. He had forgotten to secure his throttle at full military power and the force of the catapult shot had pulled the throttle back to idle. Once the force of the cat shot had subsided, he rammed the throttle as far forward as he could. I watched with riveted attention. His aircraft shot a rooster tail of ocean spray out behind him as he clawed his way skyward, avoiding death by inches as his aircraft danced over the top of the waves.

This book will rivet your attention as well. From the insights Rich offers about his addictive behavior, to the wisdom gained in dealing with his anger, to an insightful chapter concerning honesty, this book will speak to you. So strap in! *The Silent Battle* is definitely a thrilling ride!

IN THE BEGINNING

How many of us have picked up a book that begins with, "In the beginning…?" Do we really understand the meaning of "In the beginning?" In the Bible, the book of Genesis is the beginning of a great story of what life is to be like, including how and why we were created. Genesis 1:27 (NIV) says, *"So God created mankind in his own image, in the image of God he created him; male and female, he created them."* It is not by coincidence God created us to be like Him. The tough part is living by God's Word.

We were born innocent; all we could do is rely on the love and care from our parents. Unfortunately, there is no manual for parents on how to do this, how to care for their children. Many books are available with information that will help us get by in life, but what are we really looking for? Are we just looking to get by? Or are we seeking to live the way that God intends us to live? Only one book, only one truth, and one map gives us hope and direction. The Bible is a book of love stories prepared for us by God as a road map for life. Not only does the Bible prepare us for what lies ahead, but it also gives plenty of guidance for arriving there as men and women of integrity.

We all desire to live a great life. But what is life without the presence of Christ? We may have all the money, all the toys, and all the friends we could ever want or need, but let me tell you from experience, there will always be a hole to fill. You can't just stuff more money or more toys into that hole. The only way to fill the void is to invite Christ into your heart. I can tell you, however, that once you invite Jesus Christ in, your life will change forever. Nobody said living a life for Christ would be easy. We all have a target on our back, and the enemy will always try and find a way to get to you. Once you are living a life for Christ, your target gets bigger. The enemy wants nothing more than to go after one of God's own. We are called to God; He loves every one of us and has a unique call on our lives. He designed us to have a warrior spirit. We must stand hand-in-hand with God. We are all called to be conquerors in Him. There is nothing better than to go into battle with the very men who have been beaten and bruised by everyday life. The souls of men are at stake, and the Lord has called us to fight together.

We cannot fight the battles alone. Doing things on our own—without God and without other warriors around us—has caused pain in ourselves and in the lives of others around us. If we choose to continue to battle alone and not reach out for help, we will live a life of constant struggles and failure.

I hope that you find this book helpful. I pray that you will find freedom from whatever vice has a hold on you and that your true warrior within will be revealed.

God Bless!
Rich

CHAPTER 1

A SILENT BATTLE

I learned very early in life that I would have to be a fighter. I learned how to fend for myself and to get away with things. While growing up I began to seek answers to some questions that puzzled me. Why did my parents divorce after I was born? Was I the cause? Typical questions a youngster would ask. I never understood until recently how and why my path was scribed before I knew what I wanted to do in life.

It all started when I was about four years old. I was sexually molested by a trusted family member. I remember being scared, but not sure what to make of it. Was this my fault? Did I do something wrong? Was this okay with God? Right away, filled with a sense of betrayal and shame, I felt the need to take things into my own hands. I chose to live a life of secrecy and for a four-year-old, that is not the place and time to start venturing out on your own. My agenda had one thing on it: get what I thought was due me, no matter the cost. At the time I didn't know that was what I was doing, but it is obvious to me now. I learned very early in life that there were ways I could get back at people. I mastered the art of lying at a very young age. I lied so much about everything I began to believe the lies. Crazy, isn't it? I tried to blame things on other kids at school or friends in the neighborhood just so I wouldn't get in trouble. Along with the lying came another powerful behavioral choice. By the time I was five or six years old, I began stealing. I truly believed that as long as I was stealing money and toys from friends and family and lying about it, I would be fine. In my mind, it made sense that those things were owed to me because of the abuse. This continued for many years.

As I grew older and started to mature, my fantasy life soon became so overpowering that I could not function. By the age of fourteen, I was a full-blown sex addict. Along with an out-of-control fantasy life, I had become more daring when I was stealing. With my friends, I took things from the stores. I stole money from whomever and wherever. I had multiple addictions going on at the same time. I was feeding one addiction with another, falling deeper and deeper into its trap.

I became the worst version of myself at the age of fourteen; I was out of control and living deep in sexual fantasy. When the opportunity was there, I took advantage of it and violated another person. I did the same thing to her that was done to me; I sexually abused my niece (my brother's daughter). She was four years old at the time. I remember telling myself, "What am I doing? I'm going to get in trouble." As much as I told myself to stop and wanted to stop, this happened five more times. Each time the same thing happened. I told myself, "I can't do this anymore." But I was so scared and couldn't ask for help because I knew I was going to be in big trouble. Finally, I made it stop. By the grace of God she was my only victim. Nevertheless, since I was a teenage boy and so amped up sexually, I had to find other means to cope.

Two things I did well growing up—sports and my secret fantasy life. I loved baseball and was very good at it. I always believed that as long as I was pitching, I was in control and no one could stop me. At many games this was true. I had games where I struck out eleven, sixteen, even eighteen batters and pitched many complete games. I aspired to play professional baseball. That dream is still part of me. Alongside of being a good athlete in all sports, I kept and hid my secret life from those around me. Many times, I would lie about where I was going when I intended to be with a certain girl. Sometimes nothing sexual would happen; just being in the presence of a girl was enough. It made me feel like a man. And for a teenage boy, that was great! I felt I had things under control: good athlete, close female friends, and a secret no one would ever know about.

Many young guys grow up watching their siblings and try to follow everything they do. That was me. I always wanted to be just like my older brother: a great athlete, playing football and baseball, and have all the friends he had. I wanted to hang out with him even though there would be times I would get creamed in the backyard playing football or get a broken nose from playing wiffle ball. It didn't matter. I was with my older brother. The times he did not want me around, I got upset. But as long as he was at home in the yard with his friends, I was able to join, with the potential injury of course, and that was okay. My brother was there and that was all I needed and wanted.

Growing up, one of the hardest things for me to watch was my brother drive off to college. He received a full-ride scholarship to play football. The person that I felt most safe with and could always count on to be there was gone. The word "hero" is a big word and takes on a lot of meanings, but he really was my hero. There was and still is something about him that will always make him my hero.

As hard as it was to see him drive away, my life soon became much harder. By the time I reached high school, I was totally out of control. I wish I could have talked to someone. But I was too afraid of the consequences I knew would come because of what I had done to my niece. So I kept my secret. Some say that high school should be the best time of your life. And, to some extent, I would agree. But it was very challenging for me. I hid behind sports; I was a good guy with a dark secret. I was a "yes" man. I would always volunteer to help out just to make myself look good. I thought I could overcome my deep addictions by doing well in sports and helping people.

During this time I had been going to church, not much, but I knew God and had a relationship with Him, even though the relationship was one-sided. It was on my terms—when I needed Him, not when He called me. It had to be on my terms because I believed God would leave me just like my father left my mother, and like my brother left me for college. If I got too close, I reasoned, He would leave me as well, and I just couldn't handle another loss.

The crazy thing is that God's Word tells us: *No one will be able to stand against you, all the days of your life. As I was with Moses, so I will be with you; I will never leave you nor forsake you.* (Joshua 1:5 NIV) God made this promise to Joshua in preparation for what was to come. So we do not need answers to the questions that life has for us. What we need to know is that with God, all things are possible. A lot easier said than done, I assure you. I knew He would always be there for me, but I continued to sink deeper and deeper into my addictive behaviors.

I remember the first bar I entered when I was sixteen years old. Because I looked much older than sixteen, I did not get carded and neither did my friends. We thought, "This is great!" Girls all around and lots of alcohol. Once I started working and making a little money, we hit all the bars that would let us in. Pretty soon it became apparent that this was the life I wanted and I would do anything to keep coming back. This was the beginning of a lifestyle choice that would last until I turned twenty-one. For four or five years, I did whatever I could to get money, go drink, and watch the dancers. As sick as it was, I was so immersed in this lifestyle, I could not get out. As I got older and started making more money, we would go out every Friday. I spent nearly every penny I earned the prior week just for that quick fix. Sex was my drug of choice. No one knew and I was going to do everything in my power to keep it that way, and I did for many years.

At first, I thought I had everything under control; I was watching my bank account so as not to overdraw and making sure I had enough for gas to get back and forth to work. I felt consumed by a lifestyle that felt fun and acceptable until it started causing me more problems. I would call in sick for work because I stayed out too late. I had to find ways to get money so I could go back to the clubs. Not only was I bringing myself down, but also my friend who joined me. I felt bad about dragging him along with me, but I guess I didn't want to do this alone. In reality, I was alone. I had no one to confide in; I did not want anyone too close to me, except for the people at the clubs. As long as I had money, there was always something going on and I had to do whatever I could to keep it going.

For a while I went from job to job, looking for a better schedule with more pay, so I could go out more. During this time, just going to the clubs was not enough. I began to hang out with some of the girls we went to watch. I knew this was dangerous territory, but I was willing to try. This behavior continued for a few years with no one knowing. I was great at hiding behind my stature and always stayed busy doing something. That way I would never be exposed. Well, at least that was what I thought.

Just after I turned twenty-one, things started to unravel. One night I had been out late and came home wasted. I drank for hours and do not remember how or when I got home. I do remember my car was there and I was shocked that I made it. The next morning I could barely walk and was still pretty smashed. I remember going to East Hill Church in Gresham, Oregon, where I often went as a child. On that day, when Dr. Ted Roberts started talking about his own struggles with alcohol and sex addiction, I sobered up real quick. I remember walking out of church feeling like a different man. And I was.

That sermon changed me. I got involved with the church, helping out with the high school group. I continued to coach baseball and basketball, which I had been doing for a few years already. I wanted to make a difference in the lives of others and do what I could to become a man of integrity. I felt the need to give back in any way I could. I became a "yes" man again. I volunteered; if anyone needed anything, I would try to help and do the best I could. I finally felt great! Yet, even while going to church and being a part of so many positive things, I still had this battle going on inside of me. I stopped going to clubs. Thanks to God! But things were really eating at me inside. I started having anxiety attacks. I hid my emotional and mental pain from everyone. I figured, as long as I could keep doing good things, I would be able to beat this on my own. While I knew that I couldn't do things without Christ, I continued to try. Although I was helping out with the high school group, I started feeling like the fake I was and it did not feel right. I began to think of all the people who would be hurt by my behaviors and the ones I did hurt. I was about as selfish as you could get. Only one thing mattered and that was me. As long as I was okay, everything was okay.

In August of 1996, after finding my way partially back to a healthy lifestyle, I got married. I figured things were getting better; I didn't drink and I wasn't struggling sexually. I was in a healthy relationship. At least that is what I told myself. But I still had secrets. That summer was the beginning of the longest journey of my life as my mistakes and failures soon began to come to light. Proverbs 28:13 (NIV) is a powerful verse I knew and thought about frequently: *Whoever conceals his sins does not prosper, but the one who confesses and renounces them finds mercy.*

Mercy. For what I did, I told myself, who would forgive me? Who would even want to be around me if they really knew me? *Mercy.* What does that really mean anyway? The definition of mercy is offering kindness and compassion. Another is "absolution." This means forgiveness.

It was in the summer of 1996 that I was confronted with what I had done to my niece years before. I knew this was going to be a crossroads. I had two possible choices: deny and cover up or confess everything. The right thing to do is usually the hard thing to do. And that is exactly what I did. I made the decision to finally come clean about what was killing me inside. I had to come clean and face my brother, the very person I respected and trusted the most in my life. I had many emotions running through me that day. I was scared; I knew the consequences of my actions. I was scared my brother would never talk to me again. I had single-handedly put a huge amount of stress on my family and, to make things worse, I had gotten married and did not tell my wife. It wasn't long before I had a difficult conversation with my wife regarding what I had done those many years ago. We had just found out she was pregnant. Now she had a choice to make—stay or go. She made the choice to stay.

The months that followed brought immeasurable stress in my life. During this time I started attending a Pure Desire *For Men Only* group at East Hill Church. This men's group met weekly to talk about the struggles of sexual addiction. I was extremely nervous at my first meeting. These guys met early in the morning at a local pizza place. I watched and listened to these men as they shared their stories and described how they had won many battles toward sexual purity during the week. I watched them cry together and saw the empathy among them for what they had done to their families.

As I listened to their stories, I did not hear a story like mine. They all had issues, but no one had abused a child. When it came time to share my story, I started talking and focused on a couple guys I knew to try and maintain my composure; I just lost it. The floodgates opened. My eyes filled with tears as I began to reveal my story, my life. I told them how I was abused as a child; I told them I had done the same thing to my niece; I told them about the clubs, the drinking and the girls. I must have talked for fifteen minutes. I remember being scared that when it was all said and done, they would treat me differently, especially because of the abuse, but they didn't. One guy, who is still a great friend to this day, stood up, approached and hugged me, told me he was sorry, and that he loved me. I will never forget that day. He was probably the one guy, in addition to Dr. Ted, who I thought cared enough to be my friend. As I continued in this group, I experienced a new level of intimacy with Christ and a new level of friendship with the men in this group. I discovered what accountability looks like.

I knew this journey would not be easy. The Pure Desire meetings were very hard for me even though I knew I was working on my healing. Also, legal issues were now surfacing, and I was trying to do my best for my family. Proverbs 17:20 (NLT) made sense to me, especially since I was living it out so clearly: *The crooked heart will not prosper; the lying tongue tumbles into trouble.* Well, that just about covered it for me. I was a compulsive liar, I stole money, and I was a sex addict. *What else could be wrong with me?* I thought. I was really messed up. I remember my friend in the Pure Desire men's group told me it would be okay to keep coming to the group. He was right. I kept showing up, week after week, and these guys kept pouring encouraging words into my life. This was the beginning of the rest of my life. I finally found the first steps that would get me on track.

Soon after starting with the Pure Desire men's group, I had to go before the judge and face what I was certain would be many years in prison. Even though I was a minor at the time I sexually abused my niece, I was still looking at approximately thirty-six years in prison. My lawyer suggested a plea bargain, which would reduce the sentence to twenty-four years. Well, let me tell you what God had in store for me. I stood before the judge, prepared to face the consequences head on. When he handed down my sentence, I just about passed out. I was shocked! He sentenced me to ten years of probation and ninety days of work release. No prison time. That's right, no prison time. I was completely overwhelmed. God cared about me so much that He gave me another chance and spared me from prison. Talk about a merciful God!

I love 1 Timothy 1:15-17 (NLT):

> *This is a trustworthy saying, and everyone should accept it: "Christ Jesus came into the world to save sinners"—and I am the worst of them all. But God had mercy on me so that Christ Jesus could use me as a prime example of his great patience with even the worst sinners. Then others will realize that they, too, can believe in him and receive eternal life. All honor and glory to God forever and ever! He is the eternal King, the unseen one who never dies; he alone is God. Amen.*

I cannot describe how these powerful words make me feel. I felt like the worst of the worst. I had committed the most severe sin of all. But God chose me, He handpicked me, He pulled me out of the fire and breathed new life in me.

With this new start in life, I was able to get the help I needed. For the next seven years of court-ordered treatment, I took over twenty polygraph tests among other tests. Weekly, I participated in both my Pure Desire men's group and my treatment program. This was an extremely difficult time for my family. My wife and I were expecting our son in July 1997. While trying to support a family, paying for treatment, and working a dead-end job, the only thing I could do was look to God. And He came through many times. If I needed work, it was there; if we needed food, we had it. Many times we had to "rob Peter to pay Paul" as the saying goes, but we seemed to get by and had just enough. Two years later, in December 1999, we had a baby girl. I was truly blessed to have such wonderful children.

A few years later, when some issues caused conflict in our marriage, we tried to work them out. But out of my wounds, I chose to file for divorce. I thought there was nothing I could do and nothing was going to work. I loved my children deeply, but did not want them to grow up seeing my wife and I argue all the time. There were times I had second thoughts before the divorce was final, but I just kept running. I could tell I was on the verge of acting out old habits; I wanted to drink and go out to party. By the grace of God, I was still on probation. With God and the fact that I had to report once a month and take polygraph tests, I did not go back to a party lifestyle. As much as I wanted to return to that old way of life, I stayed away. For a while, I was doing alright. After I divorced, I met a few women and began some short-lived relationships that were very similar to my party days, just without the alcohol and clubs.

As hard as the divorce was on everyone—me, my wife and our children—I truly believed this was the best choice. I knew that it would be very hard on my children. While on probation, I had to have court-approved supervised visits. I was not able to see them as much as wanted. I prayed for both of my children daily and asked God to heal their hurts and help them to get through this tough period.

It took some time, but God was working on me. He started to rebuild me from the inside out. There were nights I could not sleep. I was experiencing some severe pain, but never went to the doctor. I fought through every day just to make it. During this time, I had told myself I never wanted to get married again. I was still on probation and faced an uncertain future. On a daily basis, as I walked around, I felt all alone. I told myself, *If they only knew me, really knew me, they would not like me.* These thoughts continued while attending my Pure Desire group. I knew the guys in the group liked and accepted me, but I worried about what everyone else would think. After all, I was a registered sex offender walking among them.

A few years later, I was attending a service at East Hill Church and noticed a woman sitting near my usual seat. I didn't think much about her at first, but soon made the move to go over and sit closer. I told myself I would sit over there since I had a friend that was already over there anyway; it made me feel better about my choice. During the meet-and-greet time following worship, I talked to this woman a bit. This went on for a few weeks and the conversations between us progressed to a deeper level. A few weeks later, we walked out after service together and discovered we had parked next to each other. I got up the nerve to ask her out. Funny thing about our first date, I had told her I was playing in a softball tournament at Delta Park in Portland, Oregon, and asked her to come and watch me play. To my surprise, she accepted the invite. She sat through every game I played. This made me feel great, especially since it seemed she liked sports. I thought to myself, "Cool, this can work!"

We started dating; about a year and a half later we were married. As I stated before, I never wanted to get married again, but there was just something about her. This time, before we married, I told her what I had done and that I was on probation—not an easy conversation. I really liked her, and knew I needed to be upfront about my past so she could be aware of what she was walking into. Early on in our relationship she wrote me a simple note with a quote and a verse: "*A friend is someone who comes in when the whole world has gone out*" and Proverbs 17:7 (NIV): *A friend loves at all times*. Twelve years later, I still have the sticky note she wrote to me in my Bible. She was right, if you think about it. Your true friends are always there for you, no matter what you are going through.

Things seemed to be going well, but I still had some battles going on that no one knew about. This time they were the financial kind. I had struggled with money my entire life: I hid it, stole it, lied about how I got it, and lied about where I spent it. This soon became a huge issue in my marriage. I never wanted to go through another divorce, so I tried hard to figure out how to make things seem like they were alright. I was still a compulsive liar and lied about stupid things, like getting something to eat for lunch. In our sixth year of marriage, my financial struggles came to a head. My own selfish act of stealing money from my employer created a situation in which I lost a job and I was facing legal action. I could not believe I had done this again; I had single-handedly crushed my family again. This was not the first time I had taken money while being married. I had also taken money out of my wife's account without her knowing. When all this came out, I was scared; once again I had to face the reality and consequences of my actions. I again faced the judge, but this time for theft. I was looking at a maximum ten-year sentence.

Scared that I was going to lose everything all over again, I looked to God. Only this time, He had a different lesson for me to learn. At sentencing I was certain I would get some jail time and I did. I received thirty days in jail. I thanked God for sparing me one more time. Though I was not happy about going to jail, this was the very thing that I needed in my life.

While in jail, I began to daily feast on the Word of God. After all, I had plenty of time. I asked God many times to get me out early, but He answered my prayers in a much different way. I was held in the main jail for about six days where I was celled with two other men. We started talking and they saw me reading my Bible; soon we were talking about what I was reading. I had told one of the guys who was facing thirty years in prison, "You may never experience freedom again, freedom outside the confines of the prison walls. But you can experience a new freedom that most people who are not incarcerated never experience." I told him, "You can be a warrior for Christ and fight the battle of addiction within the walls of the facility where you are going. You can do great things for the Kingdom." Later that night he began to sing a worship song he had written before he got in trouble. As he sang, I was lying in bed with the sheet over my face and began to weep. I think he met Jesus face-to-face that night. I pray that he will become that mighty warrior and fight the good fight for the men who cannot fight alone.

This is just one story about the encounters I had while in jail. I can't say I liked being incarcerated, but I must say that God had a plan and He used me to reach men who needed to hear they are loved and accepted by Jesus Christ. Most of these guys feel hated by society, as I did. What I now realize is that I am here for the purpose of Christ. It doesn't matter where I am—in jail or walking the streets. It doesn't matter. We are all called to the army of God to fight for men. We all fight a different battle every day, but we cannot fight the battles alone. We have to prepare for the war and understand that God has already gone before us.

My experiences in jail were significant in my life and profoundly changed me. I was on my way to healing and becoming vulnerable and transparent like never before. Once again, I began to process the shame I had caused my wife and family. Trust was a major issue for them, and I knew I had to change all the addictive behaviors in my life in order to have complete healing. I remember Dr. Ted saying that when the pain is great enough and we truly surrender, God will begin to direct our path for the battle ahead.

CHAPTER 2

TIME TO FIGHT

"Leadership, like coaching, is fighting for the hearts and souls of men and getting them to believe in you."[1] What a great statement by college football coach Eddie Robinson. Fighting for the hearts and souls of men. Often, a man can be fighting something that even the people closest to him don't know about. How sad is that? The battle may be sexual addiction, drugs, alcohol, gambling, or other issues—a battle that no man will be able to fight alone. The "alone" battle goes on and on for years until finally the man crumbles.

The Bible is very clear on preparing for battle. I cannot imagine going to war and fighting a battle for which I am not prepared. I have never been in a military war or even set foot on a battle-field. I can't imagine what it would be like sitting in a bunker all by yourself with the enemy coming down on you. Many soldiers today probably can tell us how it feels, but those who lack the actual experience cannot fully understand. However, I do have experience with the battlefield of my daily life in which I am at war with my addictions.

As I stated earlier, you will be unsuccessful fighting by yourself no matter what your battle. I love Ephesians 6:10-18 (NIV).

Finally, be strong in the Lord and in his mighty power. Put on the full armor of God, so that you can take your stand against the devil's schemes. For our struggle is not against flesh and blood, but against the rulers, against the authorities, against the powers of this dark world and against the spiritual forces of evil in the heavenly realms. Therefore put on the full armor of God, so that when the day of evil comes, you may be able to stand your ground, and after you have done everything, to stand. Stand firm then, with the belt of truth buckled around your waist, with the breastplate of righteousness in place, and with your feet fitted with the readiness that comes from the gospel of peace. In addition to all this, take up the shield of faith, with which you can extinguish all the flaming arrows of the evil one. Take the helmet of salvation and the sword of the Spirit, which is the word of God.

And pray in the Spirit on all occasions with all kinds of prayers and requests. With this in mind, be alert and always keep on praying for all the Lord's people.

What a powerful example of the love God has for us! He is telling us we can be victorious in our battles. Yes, we do need others around us, but we also need to arm ourselves with the Word of God. It is far more important to be fully protected by Christ than to venture out on our own. The sad thing is that every day many of us go out to face the battle without being adequately armed.

We may not all share the same battles, but we do fight the same enemy who strives to get his hooks in us. And that is exactly what he will do if we give him the opportunity. He will come at us in full force at our jobs, in our relationships, and through our finances. Wherever he can, he will try to get us. We have to be willing to be warriors and not be afraid to fight.

When I began to start seeing the battle plan unfold, I got a little nervous. A few years back, Dr. Ted had asked me to share my testimony at the church. At first I thought he was crazy, then I became overwhelmed with emotions. I started to write my story and almost instantly felt the enemy was attacking me. It was a very unpleasant feeling. I was scared! I worried that the people who would hear my story would turn away and reject me. After all, there had never been a testimony like this before in the church. People had shared their stories about drugs, alcohol, and other things. But no one had ever announced to the world (that's the way it felt to me) that they were a sex offender. After each of the five services that weekend, people stood and clapped. I saw tears in the eyes of many men, reflecting the pain they were experiencing; the same pain and hopelessness in others that I had carried for so long. Standing up and telling my story in church helped prepare me for the battles ahead.

I want to know that when my time comes and I have fought the good fight, that I have given all I had to give. Leave it all out on the field. We see this in so many sporting events—athletes giving more than they thought they had to give. Could you imagine what this world would be like today if we lived life like that? Coach Vince Lombardi summed it up this way: *I firmly believe that any man's finest hour, the greatest fulfillment of all that he holds dear, is that moment when he has worked his heart out in a good cause and lies exhausted on the field of battle—victorious.*[2]

When is the right time to fight and how do we do it? First we have to acknowledge we have a problem, like I did. When things began to unravel around me and I felt there was no hope and no one to talk to, I had but one choice. The best thing that ever happened to me was my sin being brought out into the open. This forced me to begin a healing process that will continue for years to come. If we don't realize the fight is right in front of us, then we have already lost the battle. Yes, God has gone before us and prepared the way, but if we choose not to follow His lead, we will die before we start.

Dr. Ted Roberts stated it well in his book *Pure Desire*,[3] "Our nation is getting trounced in this battle. Our moral fabric is unraveling, and the torn tapestry of people's lives is blowing in the winds of abuse, abandonment and personal trauma." This was me for years. I was headed down the path of self-destruction. I believed I had no way out. But God has a plan and when the time is right, things happen for a reason.

All men have this warrior spirit in them; we are all fighters. But what exactly is a warrior? One definition: a person who shows or has shown great vigor, courage, or aggressiveness. I have stood by some great men at East Hill Church. Great Warriors—men who will lay down everything to fight and stand in the gap for other men.

Can you imagine sitting in a bunker, having the enemy clearly in your gun site, and having no ammunition? Soldiers have their team around them—backup people who can supply more ammo and help them re-load. That is exactly what we have. We have backup. The men I have walked with for the past nineteen years have always been there when I needed them. I always knew they would be there to help me fight any battle.

So why do we have to fight so much? Sorry for the bad news! We are bombarded daily with messages contrary to godly living and healthy sexuality. Those of us who struggle with sexual addiction are especially at risk. As I drive around Portland, Oregon, I can pass a strip club or adult bookstore every ten minutes. And society says that this is okay. No wonder I was so messed up for so long. Without Christ in our hearts and men to hold us accountable, we will lose this battle against sexual addiction. There comes a point in all our lives when we have to fight. I did not want to fight at first; I was so scared of losing the battle. But in reality, I had already lost the battle when I was fighting alone!

I realized very early in court-ordered treatment programs that getting ready to fight and going into battle using tactics shared by a person who never struggled with issues similar to mine just didn't work for me. If I was going to war, I wanted to fight with men who were like me, who already had bloodstains on their clothes, who already had open wounds. These were the men I could trust. The very men I met at that first Pure Desire group. Those are the men for whom I would lay down my life.

Early on, in this battle for healthiness I told the Lord, "Please take me now if I cannot help save one child, help save one man from going down the path I chose, or help save one marriage." That is truly what I said to the Lord. Let me help just one. Many times the Lord has put men in my life who were going through some of the very things I had experienced. It was clear to me that I would be fighting for such men. The more I spoke to these men, the more I began to feel their pain. I could especially understand those who were struggling with being a registered sex offender. I soon realized that their fight was my fight as well. God was not just changing the lives of these men, but He was also changing me. I learned how to stand in the gap and intercede for them. I learned what it means to go into battle together and not alone. I learned what it takes to be a warrior for Christ, and most of all, that God trusts me with the lives of others.

You know, over 600,000 men lost their lives in the American Civil War.[4] That is just one war. Countless men have died in many wars since then—men who have fought for the freedoms we get to enjoy every day in the United States. Men lost their lives in wars they didn't necessarily believe in, but they fought because they were called to fight. They were called to be warriors and protect our nation. And that is what I strive to be—a warrior for God and His people, a warrior who will fight where needed, knowing that God is right beside me in every battle. I may never see a military war, but I am facing a war everyday in life.

Now more than ever, sexual addictions are becoming a problem in the lives of men, women, and children.[5] What better time to start than right now being a warrior for God? I have seen firsthand what happens when a man has been transformed out of his sexual addiction. I have watched as marriages are healed and lives restored. Miracles upon miracles! *Pure Desire* by Dr. Ted Roberts (the best book I have ever read) forced me to get honest with myself and learn how to fight God's way. This book helped save my life. According to Dr. Ted, we must face our own issues, no matter how painful the process. Once you choose to do this, you will undergo some very painful experiences in your healing. But you know something? The pain is worth it.

"No pain, no gain" is a saying that has been around a long time that speaks to this truth. How was I ever going to get better and experience what God has for my life if I was not willing to accept my consequences and walk through the painful healing? This is why I love sharing with other men. I love telling them my story; I love letting them know that I can walk alongside them and pray for them.

We all have things in our lives we need to change, some more difficult than others. And we all have the ability to fight. We have to fight, or we will lose to the enemy. I used to pray and hope God would take care of things. Have you ever done that? Have you ever had any unanswered prayers? All of us have. And those unanswered prayers are from God. If He simply made it easy on us and said, "Here you go, no problem," would we learn anything? No! When you choose to fight, He will start to prepare you for the battle ahead. He won't do it all for you; you have some choices to make and actions to take. However, He will give you the tools you need to make it through. The Bible is full of those tools.

This lifelong battle has its rewards. It forces me to get on my knees and spend time with the Lord. It creates a relationship with Him I can always count on. I know He is with me when I am fighting. I know He has my best interest at heart. Shame will keep you isolated, telling you daily that no one will battle with you, that you alone, and that your sin is one that will never change. Don't believe the lies of the enemy! Pick up the Sword of Truth and get in the fight.

Remember: He has chosen you and me. He knows your name and He knows your heart. We are all uniquely qualified to lead others into battle. There is no greater call than to be a warrior for Christ. What a picture—the Lord leading us into battle. We may not see Him, but He is leading us every day as we prepare for the battles we will face. Knowing He will always be there to guide my every step encourages me. He has handpicked me to battle alongside other men. What could be better than getting the call from God to fight for and with men just like me?

Lord, give me the strength to continue the battle. Help me to be a vessel for your work. I pray that you will reach the heart of every man who has a struggle that they are keeping hidden. I pray that it would be brought to light so we can battle together. Prepare the way for us, Lord, that we may be fighting the good fight. Give us the tools we need to be victorious. Amen.

CHAPTER 3

DRIVEN BY ANGER

Is there a button in your life that drives you to a place you do not want to go? Are there certain people who know what that button is and exactly how to push it? Do you even know why you have that button in the first place? If so, what would you name it? We all have those days when our button is pushed; we seem to be angry at the world and we cannot figure out why. I would challenge you to explore what pushes your anger button. Why is it so easy for us to go from one extreme emotion to the next? Are we hiding something? Tough questions!

A gentle answer turns away wrath, but a harsh word stirs up anger. The tongue of the wise adorns knowledge, but the mouth of the fool gushes folly. The eyes of the LORD are everywhere, keeping watch on the wicked and the good.

PROVERBS 15:1-3 (NIV)

How many times have I continued to say and do things that I know would just perpetuating the situation and cause some sort of "discussion?" If you are like me, guys, and most of you are, we have all had these so-called "discussions." The majority of the time I have tried to hide or deny something I did not want to deal with. So what do we do? Well, we do what we do best—shoot down the very person to whom we are married, with whom we are in a relationship, or whom is in our family. If we blow up in an angry outburst, we hope that the problem won't be brought to light. Many times, I have shot down my wife with my words because I feared what might be exposed. Because I knew I was wrong, I didn't want her to know what was going on. A marriage isn't supposed to work that way. But I can tell you that we do this out of our own insecurities and as a reaction to our own pain from the past.

I can't continue that pattern anymore. As I continue to grow in my walk with the Lord, I have learned new ways of loving and honoring my wife. I know I want to honor and love her, but is this what I do? No! I am sure you have also heard these four words that send shivers down my spine: "We need to talk." The four words I hate to hear because I know I have not loved and honored my wife the way God intends. I have ignored His Word. Why is this so difficult? I have such deep issues involving anger that it's no wonder I have shot down those around me.

As I mentioned in Chapter 1, as a victim of childhood sexual abuse, it was not by my choice that I was exposed to things a child should never know. I remember many times growing up that I would just see red. Let me explain. For me, red was not just a color, it was tied to some deep wounds and emotional trauma. Despite this, I don't recall too many outbursts of rage during my early childhood years. I would get upset and want to scream, but instead, I held my anger and rage inside. I believed that what happened to me was my fault and I was extremely angry for letting it happen. My anger even scared me. I learned to harness my anger into positive things like sports. While participating in sports I could let my feelings out without anyone knowing that my energy actually came from the anger locked away inside.

By the time I entered high school, I was already a full-blown sex addict with major anger and alcohol issues. I thought that I could handle anything. I figured that as long as my secret life was kept a secret, then everything would be fine. I also struggled with relationship issues. I never had a "girlfriend"—and not because I didn't want one. It was just that I was living a secret life and I didn't want anyone to know about. I knew a lot of girls growing up, but I thought we were just good friends and I didn't want to ruin a friendship. Looking back over the years, I have often wondered how my life would be different if I had experienced a healthy boyfriend/girlfriend relationship with one of these girls. I have recently realized that I had much more respect for the girls I grew up with than I had for myself. Now, I understand how this contributed to my use of alcohol, the club scene and unhealthy relationships very early in my teen years.

Why was I so angry with myself? Sometimes I ask myself the same question. I think it's because I never gave myself the chance to experience a healthy relationship. I had been deeply rooted in an addiction that I could not get out of, even though I wanted so badly to escape. It literally drove me nuts. I would get so angry with myself when I was out at the clubs that I would drink too much and didn't care with whom I went home. As much as I wanted to hang out with the girls I grew up with, I knew deep inside it would destroy any type of friendship I had with them. Many times, I remember seeing them with their boyfriends in school; when they would break up and get upset, I felt something happen inside me that made me very angry.

Growing up I often felt like a machine; not fully in control of my emotions, with anger as my default setting. My one purpose was to do whatever possible to retaliate. I mentioned previously about stealing and lying. What fueled that? My anger; I hated everything I stood for. I let my anger get out of control, and soon it was the driving force of my addictions; my sexual addiction and drinking became more problematic. It was like being on autopilot toward self-destruction.

Although I had already abused my niece, by the grace of God I made it out of high school without hurting another girl. God was always there, even though I was not looking for Him and really wanted nothing to do with Him. I don't think I had ever been so angry with anyone as I was with God. He said He would be faithful to us, but I didn't feel it. I felt the opposite. I believed He betrayed me and set me up. I felt like an unwanted child and thought God was embarrassed by me. At times, I even thought God was a joke.

I love my family dearly. Sometimes I have a hard time sleeping at night, still so angry over what I did to my niece. Not just her, but the impact it had on the entire family. She will always have the memory of the abuse. I can't tell you how badly I feel. Angry, oh yes! There was a time several years ago I was so upset about the direction my life had taken, I figured the best thing to do was to end it all. I got in my car, drove down to the Sandy River and parked across the street from a steep cliff that led down to the river below. I had played this event out in my mind probably a hundred times and believed this was the only way out since the pain was so unbearable. My anger had led me to what I thought was my final resting point. I waited for cars to go by for about an hour, started my car and was ready to drive off the cliff. I punched the gas pedal to the floor. The car started to go, but then died. I was so mad, I began to cry. I just wanted to die. This was too much for me to handle. I never told anyone. Again, I felt like such a failure, I couldn't even kill myself. God obviously intervened—again. I could not understand what He wanted with me. I was a wreck; a big disappointment.

Once I was out of high school and working, things seemed to calm down a bit. I still had secrets, but somehow managed to get by; although, getting by on my standards, often meant not making the best choices. I brought all my issues into the marriage with my first wife. She didn't have a chance. I had sabotaged our relationship before we even met. During this time I was on probation, which was very difficult for me. I could not tap into what was causing me to be so angry with everyone. In our relationship, my wife would push buttons that she didn't even know were buttons. The dumbest things would set me off. My anger, among other issues, led to our divorce.

Shortly after my divorce, I was at my parents' house; we were talking about my children and what I was going to do. I remember my step dad and I got into an argument that kept escalating, getting hotter and hotter. I then saw RED and for the first time, I acted on it. With extreme force, I shoved my step dad into the wall, leaving a hole in the wall. It was so strange. Even right after it happened, I didn't even remember touching him; it felt like it didn't happen. My reaction scared me. Another button pushed, maybe? Not sure. After that incident, my anger started to manifest itself in a very physical way. When I felt angry, I responded by punching holes in walls and doors. One time I hit a closet door in the hallway so hard that my arm went all the way through the door. I practically had to cut the door away just to get my arm out. I punched a wall one time, hit the stud, and just about broke my hand. Every time I felt threatened, I hit something. And it continued to get worse.

Unfortunately, I brought this behavior into my current marriage. My wife now is a strong woman and will speak her mind. She is not afraid to confront me with any issue. This is a very good thing. God really blessed me with such a great wife. It was time for me to start dealing with the anger. By this time, my alcohol abuse and the sexual addiction were pretty much under wraps.

Through this process, I have learned the root cause of my anger issues (the abuse I suffered as a child) and have continued to walking in that healing. I am able to recognize my anger triggers, but continue to work on strengthening my anger management skills on a daily basis. Just recently my wife and I had a "discussion" about finances, and, yes, she was right and I was wrong. I knew this was coming, and I did everything in my power to deny my part. I lied, raised my voice, started seeing RED again, and then turned and punched the door, putting yet another hole in something. I have lost count of the number of times this has happened. What can I say? I am a work in progress.

I like what God's Word says about anger: *My dear brothers, take note of this: Everyone should be quick to listen, slow to speak and slow to become angry, for man's anger does not bring about the righteous life that God desires* (James 1:19-20 NIV).

One way I have learned to manage my anger is to turn it into something good. The tough part for me is having a split second to make the choice to turn the anger to something positive; nine times out of ten, I have failed miserably. When I come face-to-face with issues I know will cause some sort of argument, I fail. Some time ago my wife asked me how I spent my money. When I told her what I spent it on, she had a hard time believing me; she remembers the times I lied to her about finances. I became very angry and could have made things worse, but instead I told myself I needed a timeout. The "timeout" is a great gift, I think created by God, and so useful when I'm starting to boil. Don't think you can do it on your own. I am living proof that our sins will always rise to the surface; they will find a way to come to the light. Timothy Light, a man who experienced extreme loss and grief, expresses it well:

> *Anger hides in the bowels of the soul stealing energy that can be used for positive feelings.*
>
> *Such an easy feeling to portray, the hardest to control.*
>
> *Anger is like a desert wind picking up sand and hurling it toward an unsuspecting being causing pain. The mind goes numb.*
>
> *Existence is meaningless. Actions are uncontrollable.*
>
> *Repercussions do not exist. Anger takes over the body and sends it into a violent rage.*
>
> *Thoughts may be twisted. Nightmares come at night.*
>
> *The demon has taken control.*
>
> *Sorrow for the anger washes across the body feels pain.*
>
> *The mind feels numb. Such a horrible process. Show the love.*[6]

The first two lines say it all. Read it again to yourself, and then read it out loud. Listen to what the words are saying. I don't know your reaction, but the very first line sounds like the devil lurking, waiting for us to slip up. When anger clouds our judgment we can make terrible decisions, sometimes requiring weeks or months to repair the damage and earn back the trust. While anger is often a good sign that something is truly wrong, it is important to carefully consider how you will respond. You may need to process other emotions and ask the Lord for His perspective.

After years of struggling with my anger, I still believed that everything would be fine because I had finally disclosed my sexual addiction. I was good, all healed. Wrong! My anger was now triggered by being questioned when my behaviors did not match with my words.

Be angry, and do not sin; ponder in your
own hearts on your beds, and be silent.
PSALM 4:4 (ESV)

For the evildoers shall be cut off, but those who wait
for the LORD shall inherit the land.
PSALM 37:9 (ESV)

A fool gives full vent to his anger,
but a wise man keeps himself under control.
PROVERBS 29:11 (ESV)

Get rid of all bitterness, rage and anger, brawling
and slander, along with every form of malice.
EPHESIANS 4:31 (NIV)

CHAPTER 4

THE PAIN OF BETRAYAL

When I started to outline the chapters of this book, I knew I would have to add a section on betrayal. I want to define it in a way that will help you understand the pain it creates. I hope that as you read this, guys, you can visualize where you were when you were not doing well and see how your actions betrayed and impacted others.

I asked my mom to write this chapter as she was so deeply hurt by my betrayal and by the tearing apart of our family. Here are her words:

BY KATHY WIGLE, MY MOM

I remember the very day my son's life changed, but I didn't have a clue why. He was such a wonderful four-year-old, full of life and fun. I was always amazed at how well behaved and well adjusted he was, even though in his four short years I had gone through a divorce and remarried.

At first, I noticed little things and then began to see him get more angry with every passing day. Things would show up missing or his brother would have something missing from his room and Rich would cry and say, "I didn't do it" and we believed him. At the time, I didn't know that my son was suffering the effects of being sexually abused. The anger, lies, and stealing would continue for years.

The sting of betrayal is something I had experienced in my previous marriage. I was separated from Rich's dad for most of my pregnancy and divorced by the time Rich was two months old. I understood what it felt like to have your spouse go through multiple affairs and also be an alcoholic on top of it. I had to leave my new baby and return to work to support him and his brother. This was the life of a single mother. My only thought was to raise my children and do the best I could by them, keeping them safe and helping them walk through this difficult time. *"We have this hope as an anchor for the soul, firm and secure. It enters the inner sanctuary behind the curtain, where Jesus, who went before us, has entered on our behalf."* (Hebrews 6:19-20 NIV) Our anchor is only as secure as that to which it is fastened. I began to anchor myself in Christ; He was a safe place for me. He understood the betrayal and shame I was facing because He experienced it. Jesus was betrayed by his closest friends and suffered the shame of the cross.

When I went to work for Dr. Ted Roberts at East Hill Church, I had no idea that God was equipping me for what was about to take place in our family. I was a staff pastor at East Hill Church for fourteen years and had a chance to help many women walk through the betrayal that they felt in their marriage, caused by affairs and/or sexual addiction. I could be empathetic because of what I had walked through in my own personal experience. I had no idea what was to come!! I would soon learn that my son was a sex addict and his struggles were severe.

When Rich met with the whole family and confessed what he had done, I thought my life was over. I was angry, hurt beyond words, and so confused. I blamed myself, God, and everyone else I could think of. The betrayal cut like a knife into my soul. Everything I believed in was gone in an instant. Listening to my son tell his story was like listening to someone who was a total stranger. Looking back now, I can begin to put the pieces of his life together from the time he was abused at age four. I felt betrayal all over again. Not only by Rich, but also because I believed I had totally abandoned him; I never knew about the abuse. I realized that this was the start of his downward spiral into addiction. As he confessed to what he had done, everything I knew to be true in my life was shattered. My pain, guilt, and shame were so deep that I didn't think I would ever be the same again. I knew the answer, but it felt like God was there for everyone else but my family and me. After all, I worked at the church and I helped people. What would people think if they knew?

God seemed very far away. The more I prayed, the more the enemy tried to convince me it would never change. I wanted to believe that God could fix this, but I felt only emptiness. I was battle weary. The future was so uncertain. I didn't want to face what people would be saying about my son. I was filled with anger and shame, not only towards Rich, but also with myself. I thought, I must have missed the warning signs. I felt the sorrow of watching the victim go through difficult times of healing and counseling, and the family trying to deal with the ups and downs of an emotional roller coaster. There were times we didn't know where to turn, but God always provided someone to stand with us to give us strength when we couldn't take another step.

After Rich confessed everything that he had kept hidden for so long, I went through a two-month period of depression. I had always loved our family get-together times and the holidays, but now, the thought of it was dreadful; our family was torn apart and we couldn't all be together. There was so much pain in our family and there was no place to go to escape it. We were in the grieving stages of loss—loss of family and loss of relationship. We also had to watch our family member go through her pain of recovery. Knowing what the victim was going through made it all the more difficult to start on the road of forgiveness with Rich. How could we trust him again? Was he being honest with us? Could I open my heart again to someone I thought I knew, but really didn't? These were difficult questions to ask, and the answers didn't come for a long time. After having some counseling myself, I realized that the hardest person to forgive was me. It was difficult to understand that sex addicts are masters of manipulation and deception because they have had to keep the secret hidden away. Even if they have a commitment to Christ, they have literally compartmentalized their lives so they can carry on two lives at once—a public life and a private life, which is what Rich had been doing for years.

The road back has been long and painful, as all of us in the family have had to heal and continue healing to this day. We are not the same; we are stronger today because we have gone through the difficult storms and allowed God to change us. Each of us made a decision to step out of the betrayal and allow God to show us the path to forgiveness. We made a choice. By choosing to forgive, we were able to move past the hurt that could have taken root as bitterness and would have kept us from experiencing the healing and the new level of family that we have now.

Diane Roberts wrote an important truth in the *Betrayal & Beyond Workbook: Fashioning a Courageous Heart*: "Remember that forgiveness occurs directly between you and God first, before it can ever flow back through you to another person. It is not simply words, but is a miraculous exchange that occurs spiritually."[7] Jesus showed us how to do this when He was dying on the cross. In the midst of His agony He said, *"Father, forgive them, for they do not know what they are doing."* (Luke 23:34 NIV) He began the forgiveness process by settling the issue with God before it could ever be resolved in relationship. As He stated in John 20:23 (NIV), *"If you forgive anyone's sins, their sins are forgiven; if you do not forgive them, they are not forgiven."* He chose to use His free will to forgive us before we even knew we had offended Him because He wanted nothing to interfere in His relationship with God. Out of the freedom that comes from forgiveness, you will be able to hear God as never before. Spend some time listening to what He would say, expecting the Holy Spirit to speak to you. Journal those words that come to mind as you practice listening through prayer.

Everything about betrayal is deeply intimate. God knows that, and He is not surprised or offended when you tell Him the truth. He already knows every intimate detail of what occurred and it is for your heart's sake that you speak the truth to Him. Betrayal is shrouded in secrecy and shame. When we choose to forgive, we heal the hurt we didn't deserve. No one deserves to be hurt by others, and yet, because we live in this world, pain comes to us. Sometimes we add to the pain of the situation, but no one asks to be wounded or to be punished through great emotional, physical, and spiritual harm. Choosing to forgive releases us to begin the healing process within. It unshackles us from the wound.

I am proud of my son for having walked this most difficult path of healing. He has taught me so much about myself and also about how to love the unlovely. He has taught me that we have a gracious and loving God who reaches down into the very core of our pain. We are still on our healing journey, and excited for what God has for us in the future. *Thank you, Lord, for never leaving or forsaking my family as we have walked this healing path.* Rich and I have been strengthened as we minister to others who are walking where our family has walked in regards to sexual addiction. We see the miracle and tremendous hope of what God has done and continues to do. Being able to encourage others is walking in that healing. We have been to the depths of despair, but we have seen God change our lives and our hearts. It is not only Rich who has changed, but myself as well.

Rich and I share the same passion for the Pure Desire ministry. We didn't realize how prophetic 2 Corinthians 1:4 (MSG) would be for us: *He comes alongside us when we go through hard times, and before you know it, he brings us alongside someone else who is going through hard times so that we can be there for that person just as God was there for us.* We have experienced that comfort first hand and have been able to comfort others as the Lord has placed us in this ministry. Being able to see other families come to health and wholeness has been such a blessing to me. To see the pain of betrayal replaced by the grace and mercy of Christ as families walk through the difficult times, to begin seeing there is hope for them.

I give thanks to my Lord and Savior Jesus Christ for surrounding us with such love and support over the years. To my dear friends, Nancy and Rosemary, to Scot who loved on my husband and I during those early days of disclosure, to Pastor Harry who saw something of value in my son and walked with him in the restoration process. To the families that I have had the honor of meeting with and encouraging during the difficult journey, thank you. You have enriched my life as you have allowed me to share with you and be a part of your story. And lastly, to Dr. Ted Roberts who has been not only my boss and my friend, but also a man who has sacrificed so much to give men like Rich a hope and a future. Pure Desire Ministries saved my son's life and saved our family from total devastation. Thank you, Pure Desire Ministries International, for being there for our family during this long journey of healing.

CHAPTER 5

FORGIVENESS, MERCY, AND GRACE

One of the biggest and hardest parts of the healing journey is learning to walk in forgiveness. Continuing to not forgive those who hurt us will cause us a lot of pain. Not only are we to forgive others, but we also must forgive ourselves. How do we do that? I hope you will see in this chapter what forgiveness looked like for me and others.

Forgiveness is a much-repeated theme in the Bible. 1 Chronicles 21:8 (MSG) resonates with me:

> *Then David prayed, "I have sinned badly in what I have just done, substituting statistics for trust; forgive my sin— I've been really stupid."*

The footnotes in my NIV Bible explain that when David realized his sin, he took full responsibility, admitted he was wrong, and asked God's forgiveness. Can you imagine what that conversation was like? I can; I have had the same conversation with God.

I always knew I was messed up. I did some extremely stupid things, as you know from reading my story. For a long time I refused, absolutely refused, to ask God to forgive me because I truly believed He didn't care about me. Many times I blamed God for what I was doing and what I had done. Sad, isn't it, that we can know He will always be there for us, and yet, all we can do in return is blame Him for our problems. I didn't start experiencing true forgiveness until my sin was brought to light. New life starts with forgiving ourselves because until we forgive ourselves, we are incapable of truly forgiving others who have hurt us. And that was exactly what was wearing on me. I could not get over what I had done to my niece; it was literally killing me inside. I was completely lost and did not know where to turn. But, by the grace of God my sin was exposed. This was one of the best and most difficult times in my life. As I started walking this healing path, I realized that I had to learn how to forgive myself. I also experienced forgiveness from those I had hurt. I saw what God was doing, and then continued on the right path. But I still struggled with all that I had done. It wasn't until a few years after the abuse came out that I really felt like a different person and that I was able to make that next step. My family showed me what true forgiveness, grace, and mercy looked like.

2 Corinthians 12:9 (NIV) says, *"But he said to me, 'My grace is sufficient for you, for my power is made perfect in weakness.' Therefore I will boast all the more gladly about my weaknesses, so that Christ's power may rest on me."* I truly began to believe that the Lord was perfect in my weakness and that He could do anything in me, if I let Him—so I did.

As you read the following stories of forgiveness, grace, and mercy lived out in my family, I encourage you not only to just read the words, but also to feel their pain and think about how difficult it was for them to extend this forgiveness to me. For that I am grateful. 1 Kings 8:50 (NIV) says: *And forgive your people, who have sinned against you; forgive all the offenses they have committed against you, and cause their captors to show them mercy.*

FROM KATHY WIGLE, MY MOTHER

The process of forgiveness is illustrated by a true-life story about Corrie Ten Boom.[8] She and her family were prisoners in a German concentration camp during World War II. Being the only one in her family to survive, after the war she had to work through a lot of pain and forgiveness. One day as she walked down the street in post-war Germany, she passed by a German guard and felt intense anger suddenly welling up within her.

She thought she had forgiven the guards and was so concerned with her reaction that she immediately went to visit her pastor. After hearing Corrie's story, he led her to the bell tower of the church. He asked her to pull hard on the rope and ring the large tower bells. After she had pulled the rope many times, he told her to release it. The sound of the bells continued to reverberate through the air until they finally slowed to silence.

He told her that her decision to forgive was a releasing of the bell rope of resentment she had pulled on for so long. Ringing echoes remained even though she had released the rope. Notice the first step was the bells ringing. We have to get in touch with our "rope" of hurt, anger, and bitterness and express it in healthy ways.

When I read this story, it brought me back to the pain and resentment I felt toward my son. My "rope" of hurt and anger was so deep. How could he have had this secret life that no one knew about? After all, I was his mother and I should have caught it. As a parent, learning that your twenty-one-year-old son had been sexually abused at the age of four was one of those moments you never want to hear. On top of this revelation, the family was told that he had sexually abused a family member. I immediately went from shock to denial to extreme pain.

I love this quote by an unknown author: *I forgave to set a prisoner free, only to discover that the prisoner was me.*

Choosing to forgive allowed my heart to begin to heal. It ripped the scab of numbness off my heart and allowed God to come and cleanse the infection in that wound. Romans 12:19 (NIV) clearly states: *Do not take revenge, my dear friends, but leave room for God's wrath, for it is written, "It is mine to avenge; I will repay," says the Lord.* Only God can judge with justice.

To all who were part of our strong support system: Words can never express how much you have meant to our family. From the very beginning you were there for us, offering your prayers and encouragement—never judging. It was an overwhelming period in our lives we could not have walked through without you. The pain of maneuvering through the healing process was difficult. Hebrews 12:2 declares that Jesus endured the cross for the joy set before Him. The term "endured" has to do with courageously facing the trials and tribulations life brings because we've caught sight of something much greater than what we're going through. In the process, the difficulty is transformed by the vision that pulls us to higher ground. Forgiveness is a picture of integrity in the midst of personal pain. Both integrity under pressure and integrity in the midst of personal pain underline a deep challenge for us all because we all have a hard time forgiving.

To be a person who walks in forgiveness and who lives within God's authority, we also need to decide to walk in the blessing God has set aside for us. If we've said "yes" to Christ the Son, then God the Father has set His heart to bless us. The enemy knows that, and it deeply troubles him. He would love to get his hands on us, but in order to do so he has to get us out of the place of blessing. Forgiving is risking; for those of you reading this book, I pray you would be able to start the process of forgiving and walk in the blessings that God the Father has set before you.

Psalm 103:2-6 (NIV) is a pivotal scripture: *Praise the Lord, my soul, and forget not all his benefit—who forgives all your sins and heals all your diseases, who redeems your life from the pit and crowns you with love and compassion, who satisfies your desires with good things so that your youth is renewed like the eagle's. The Lord works righteousness and justice for all the oppressed.*

My mom's story is powerful, isn't it? Nobody ever said that forgiveness would be an easy thing; in fact, it is the exact opposite.

When my daughter was about twelve years old, I found out that she had been previously sexually molested; she was eight at the time of the incident. It immediately brought to the surface intense pain and anger. I could not believe that my own daughter had to go through this, especially since I always wanted to protect my children from any of this happening to them. Remember when I prayed that I wanted to help at least one child escape abuse? How could I do that? I couldn't even stop it from happening to my own child! I was so upset when I found out. Here I was trying to reach out to men who struggle with sexual addiction and help them to do what is right, and now, I was faced with forgiving a man who did the same thing to my daughter that I did to my niece. It is hard to describe the pain a parent feels when this happens, and some days I still have a hard time accepting that my daughter was the victim of sexual abuse. I now understand what my family had to go through. I would not want anyone to experience this pain.

My baby girl was hurt and there was nothing I could do about it. I talked with family members about how I was feeling and what they had gone through. I knew I must forgive the man who hurt my daughter, but how could I? I kept looking to God for the answers. Matthew 6:14-15 (NIV) says: *For if you forgive other people when they sin against you, your heavenly Father will also forgive you. But if you do not forgive others their sins, your Father will not forgive your sins*. I didn't want to go through life with God not forgiving me. I had always forgiven people in my life, but this was different. After all, it was my daughter. But you know what? I had a quiet conversation with God and let this man go in my heart; I released him to Jesus. I had to. It was the only way that I could help my little girl go through the healing process and not let her see the extent of my anger.

The Lord has done great things in our family and continues to do so, especially when we hit the tough times. I see new miracles every day and I see Him working in our lives. Here is another story of forgiveness. For those wives reading this, hang in there; the process is long and painful but well worth the reward that the Lord has for you.

FROM DENEEN, MY WIFE

I met my husband during his recovery process. He was truthful, honest, and up-front about his conviction. Little did I know the impact it would have on my life, since I did not know much about the recovery process for sexual addiction and addictive behavior. I began this journey with him in his recovery by attending a meeting with his court appointed behavioral counselor. Learning his guidelines and boundaries was difficult; having to watch him be accountable and answer to a probation officer once a month was not pleasant. He continued to go to his Pure Desire men's group weekly. Rich had a great group of guys around him and they helped keep him in check. By this time we had married and Rich took a job in sales. After a short time, I began to see some changes in his honesty. Rich was coming home with money almost every night, but I never knew how much; I questioned him and he always said it was delivery tips. Each time I questioned him, his answer was always the same story.

The night before I was to come home from an out-of-town job training, we spoke on the phone. Rich, sounding distraught, said he really needed to speak with me. I asked, "What is going on?" He just said, "Hurry and get home; I need you."

After Rich told me he had stolen money from his employer, I didn't want to forgive him. I felt he put me through this pain for no reason. I didn't even see it coming, so to forgive him was the last thing I was going to do. I reasoned, *This is a man of God, right? For any woman to have to go through such pain is totally unacceptable.*

He was fired from his job and a short time later he suffered the consequences of his actions—time in jail. During the time Rich was away, I continued to seek God and reach out to friends for support. One evening at church, I was struggling; I knew it was time to forgive him, but I still did not want to do that. I spoke with a great friend named Wally, and we talked about forgiveness. He told me that this was not about Rich—that it was about my relationship with Christ. I did not want to have this lack of forgiveness in my life.

Wally told me to tell Rich that I forgave him. When I stepped out in faith to forgive and spoke the words to Rich, "I forgive you," I was truly transformed. I've never looked back. My greatest joy is seeing Rich continue to help others in their journey to restoration. I see a new man that is being molded every day. Growing pains always accompany the growth, and I see the work that God is doing in his life, as well as mine.

ABOUT MY BROTHER PAT

I want to share briefly about my brother, who is the father of the niece I abused. When the abuse of my niece come out, it was extremely difficult on all of us. As time went by, I began to understand things about myself, realized why this happened and what I had to do to regain trust from the family. I knew this would not be an easy task. I never expected anything to be remotely like it was before the abuse took place. I can see now that the Lord was fighting for our family. I also now see my brother from a different perspective. The first few years after the abuse was revealed, my brother and I had very little communication; it was very challenging for both him and his wife. Yet, I knew and believed God was working. It was never my place to ask to be a part of his family after what happened. I never expected it. It took time, but we were able to create a new relationship. I will always be grateful that my brother has given me a second chance.

My brother is one of the best men I know. He showed me grace and let me back into his life when I didn't deserve it. I imagine there may be times he wonders if he has done the right thing. I see the battles he and his wife had to endure to get to where we are today. I can never repay them for what I did or go back and undo what I did. But I can move forward, follow God, and trust that He will make all things new.

When my daughter was abused, I better understood the anger, hurt, and frustration that my family, especially my brother, experienced. It takes a very strong man to forgive someone who has done the things I've done, but my brother Pat has showed me what the love of Christ looks like by his actions and the fact we are a family again. It is weird how God works. My brother having the strength to let me back into his life has brought amazing Holy Spirit healing to our family. Not a day goes by that I don't pray for my niece. Saying "I'm sorry" will never be enough to undo what I did, but I know God will help her in the same way He helped me.

As you have just read, the power of forgiveness is truly a wonderful thing. For us to move past the painful events that happen in our lives, we must absolutely forgive those who are the source of our pain. This process will never be easy for anyone. But forgiveness—both asking and receiving—allows the Holy Spirit to enter the situation and bring release and inner healing to everyone; those who forgive and those who are forgiven. We are always going to face situations in our lives that will require us to be forgiving. The same mercy and grace that the Lord has given to us, we can give in return.

Writing this book has reopened my wounds again. I am continually learning how to forgive myself. I know the gifts that God has for us are too great to pass up. If we are unable to let someone go through the process of forgiveness or to forgive ourselves, we will continue to live our lives as a hostage.

Lord, I pray that each and every person reading this today will reach a point where they can experience Your true forgiveness. Give them the strength to reach out and seek help from You. Help them to experience mercy and grace. Lord, be their Rock during their weakness. Amen.

CHAPTER 6

CROSSROADS
TO HONESTY

Honesty: A refusal to lie, steal or deceive in any way. (Webster's Dictionary)

Pretty matter of fact, isn't it? Short and to the point! I wish I could have lived out honesty early in my life. Sometimes we walk through life hiding things from other people. We hide so we can live without having to be accountable. Why? We're scared. We don't want to be embarrassed, hurt, or looked down on. We lie or hide things we do not want others to know about us—secrets, addictions, things that carry unsavory consequences. That was the case in my life for many years.

I always thought that if I could keep my secret life hidden from others, I would be able to overcome my past and be alright. And, this worked for a while; at least I thought I was alright. In reality, I could not function because I had so much garbage in my life. I was rooted deep into an addictive lifestyle that no one knew about. I hid it from everyone. I was so scared I could not even be honest enough with myself to ask for help. I knew I was going down and I did. I hit rock bottom. It wasn't until mid-1997 that I began to get honest. Not just with myself, but also with my family, friends, and, most of all, with God.

Proverbs alone contains more than twenty verses about honesty. *The LORD is more pleased when we do what is right and just* (Proverbs 21:3 NLT). The author of Proverbs doesn't say that doing right will be easy. We have a saying in our Pure Desire groups: *Doing the right thing is usually the hard thing.* And for me it was very difficult. I had to learn how to be transparent, vulnerably transparent. What does that mean? Well, I had to be accountable to men I was meeting with on a weekly basis. Not just in the meeting, but in phone calls during the week. I learned that being honest about my current situation and how I was doing enables the Holy Spirit to work in me. *He [the LORD] delights in honesty* (Proverbs 12:22 NIV). He truly loves it when we come to Him with an open and pure heart—something I had never been able to do before.

As I mentioned earlier, 1997 was a crossroads year for me. I had two choices: deny what happened or be honest and let God take it from there; take me from there. I chose God. I already knew Him, but I had my own agenda. I remember making the right decision for one of the first times in my life. My life began to change. It was not an easy road. Many others were affected by my poor choices and I knew that I had to finally face the very thing that I ran toward when I was feeling bad. I had been choosing my addiction over family, friends, and God. Once I made that right decision to choose God over my addiction, I finally was able to work on my issues. It took a long time to gain the trust of those whom I hurt and lied to for years, including myself. One of my friends told me I had to be brutally honest. I finally got it! I finally felt like there was some hope. In my very first Pure Desire group, when I told everything that I was going through and what I had done, I finally felt the enemy step back away from me. I shared things that most people would never discuss. But I knew

I had to tell it all. When I made that decision to become brutally honest, my life changed forever.

These changes did not take place overnight. It was a process. I was at rock bottom, and there was only one real answer. I knew the truth would set me free. I had gone through many years of counseling, training, and growth. I was in my late thirties now, and finally felt that I was on the right path. It was hard for those in my family, very hard for many years. But I knew that I had to get busy and do the right thing.

One book I have read many times is Stephen Covey's *The 7 Habits of Highly Effective People: Powerful Lessons In Personal Change*.[9] I learned how to set goals, short term and long term. I needed to set limits and learn how to schedule my time. Why is this book so important to me? It was the first book I read while I was in counseling. It forced me to look at my life and set some direction. It forced me to be honest with myself and learn to be productive, instead of hiding. I finally understood how to trust God and not worry about what others would think of me.

To this day, I look back and cannot believe how far I have come. God began to heal me as well as those I had hurt. I knew it was important for me to find a relationship with God in which I could tell Him everything. God gave me the tools and instilled in my heart the meanings of honesty and transparency. I did not have to hide behind my secrets any more. I could trust those around me with anything. The very thing that was destroying me became the very thing I love to do. I love when I have the opportunity to share my story with other men. My transparency and honesty give them a glimpse of hope. It lets them know it is okay to share what is wrong, what is going on in their lives. When

I share about my walk through recovery, I know that the enemy is boiling mad. God gets the glory and the devil flees when I am honest in what I do and what I speak.

The toughest part of the past twelve years is looking back on my family and the hurt I caused them. I went through a divorce and was separated from my kids for a while. I never thought a family could experience so much pain because of one person, a dishonest person! I didn't realize the impact my life would have on them. I never thought my secret life would get out and that we all would have to endure so much pain. But you know what? God took that pain and covered our family. He began working differently in each of our lives and it started with me being honest. I could have taken the wrong path and chosen to not do the right thing. But deep in my heart, I knew I must be open to what God was going to do in my life. God is truly good. As I was being honest with God, He began fulfilling the dreams of my heart. He brought me the most wonderful woman I could ever know. I never thought I would ever get married again, but I believed God had someone for me. And He did. One of the first times we talked, I told her everything about me—what I did and where I was in life. I was open and honest with her about my addiction, thinking I would never see her again after that revelation. It was soon clear that God had brought her into my life. I learned how to be honest with her in every aspect of life. And, yes, there were times it was hard, but God truly blessed me.

Blessed are the pure in heart, for they will see God (Matthew 5:8 NIV). What a great Scripture. I love the simplicity of the words. For me, a pure heart is an honest heart. No walls, no lies, no hiding. When I call on God with a pure heart, He always comes through, maybe not in the way I prayed or in my timeframe, but He always shows up. When I chose to make the right choice and get the help I needed, He showed up and guided me. He washed my slate clean. One thing I need to add here is that God is always with us; He will never leave, nor forsake us. Before, I was so blinded by my own selfish desires that I could never sense His presence or see Him work in my life.

Honesty will look and feel different for each of us. But in the end, all God asks of us is to be truthful with our words and honest with our hearts. Sometimes, it will be very difficult. And if it feels hard, you know you are doing the right thing. Jesus calls us to "*let your light shine before others, that they may see your good deeds and glorify your Father in heaven.*" (Matthew 5:14-17 NIV) Can we really accomplish the smallest of things that God asks us to do if we are not being honest with Him and others around us? I would not be where what I am today had I chosen a different path at that honesty crossroad. If you are on a road that is too easy then you are not going far. The enemy tempts us with instant gratification. Guys, it is time to get down to business and do the right thing. Not just for us, but for those who love us and are counting on us. Remember: the hard thing to do is usually the right thing to do.

Something you probably didn't want to hear—but here it is anyway: Honesty hurts at times. Have you ever lied to your spouse about where you ate lunch and how much you spent? I have. The discussions that followed were painful. It would have been so much easier had I just spoken the truth, instead of being dishonest.

We live in a society that promotes sexual, alcohol, and other addictions. There are bars on almost every corner. We are set up for failure and addiction by the enemy of our souls. So we learn to be dishonest. We learn to cover our tracks. Now guys, here is a question for you. Have you ever lied to your wife about where you were? Were you at a topless bar, out drinking with the guys, working late? And I don't mean working late at work; it is an excuse many men use as they have been involved with co-workers and who knows who or what else.

God will always be there and He delights in our honesty. (Proverbs 11:1) Are you at an honesty crossroad? What is holding you back from taking the next step? Some of those behaviors I practiced? But you know what? You can do it. You have to do it. The Lord loves each one of us. You are not alone, even though it may feel like it; He is waiting for you to fall into His arms.

It is truly an impossible task to live a life for Christ while hiding things from those around you. I tried to keep secrets from God. How messed up is that? Keeping secrets from God? Yep! That is what I did. I truly believed that my secret life was a secret. Only when I began to be honest with myself did things begin to change. At times, the old self crept in and I just wanted to hide. I'm not doing that anymore. The Lord has done remarkable things in my life and He continues to send blessings to me in ways I could never have imagined.

I could not have arrived at this point in my life without the encouragement from so many great men around me who show me what it looks like to walk in integrity and be an honest man. Mike, Harry, Ted, Pat, Scott, Wally, John, and the list could go on for pages, but I wanted to share just a few of the best men I know and love dearly. These men have been praying for me for years. There is nothing I wouldn't do for them. I have witnessed their honesty and integrity lived out in their lives. Great role models! I have learned from them the type of man I want to be—a husband, father, and friend. I hope you begin to find men of integrity and honesty to walk alongside you.

CHAPTER 7

WASHED CLEAN

A few years ago, a friend, who knew my wife and I were going through a tough time, invited me to attend a church small group. I didn't want to go, but I knew this was an appointment set up by God. Prior to the meeting, my wife and I had been struggling with our finances. We had been having those "conversations" and getting nowhere. This was a real tough financial time for us, and especially for me as a man. I could not provide for my family. I was trying to do it all and was not seeking the Lord's provision. I was still holding onto things that were bothering me; I had a resentful and unforgiving heart. But I decided to show up at the meeting anyway.

God tells us clearly in Scripture that He will never leave us, and I knew that. But to feel His presence the way I did that night was remarkable. How awesome to listen to the stories of what the guys were going through and to spend time praising God! I had been in many men's groups, but this was the next level for me. The Holy Spirit was so obviously present I could almost see Him and sensed His presence on the men's faces and in their words.

When it was my turn to share, all I could do was emotionally break down; I couldn't talk and I started crying. I felt like such a failure to my wife, my kids, and the rest of the family. I thought I could do nothing right and that no matter how good I was doing, the Lord still had forgotten about me. But God showed up that night and set me straight. As my eyes were full of tears, I felt one gentleman cup his hand under my chin as my eyes were closed; it felt like he was catching my tears and that made me cry even more. They laid hands on me, prayed for me, and just loved on me when I needed it most. I felt the hand of God. One of the guys had asked me to take my shoes and socks off, so I did. He proceeded to wash my feet. At that moment, I felt like something change in me; this was the first time I experienced a foot washing. I felt as if all my burdens were lifted and my slate had been wiped clean. There was nothing left for me to carry alone.

Until that time, I was still carrying a lot of pain from my past, especially surrounding what I did to my niece. I had watched her go through some tough times, and I was so upset knowing I was the cause of her struggles. I felt bad that she was experiencing so much pain. I know that our family has endured new growth and healing, but the pain that she has been through hurts me. Many questions plague my mind: *Would her marriage be work out? Can she trust anyone again?* Question after question! *Why, Lord, why did I have to do this to her? She did not deserve to experience the pain as I did, so why, Lord? Why couldn't You have saved her from me?* So many times I beat myself up. After all, I was family and it had been my role to keep her safe.

So why did God lift my burdens and wash my slate clean? Why did He give me a second chance? And what would end up on this new slate? As I continued on this journey the Lord set before me, I realized that many men need help. I could not do God's work or be of assistance to these guys if the Lord did not show up and wash me clean. He literally took all my pain away that night. He breathed new life into me.

A new life and new direction bring on new challenges, and they came after that night. Even though I made mistakes along the way, I now sense the presence of Christ every day. I know that He will show Himself in a sermon, a song or even in a thought. I know I can count on Him. I had never felt like this before. I have always struggled with worry. Have you ever been called a worrywart? When I was young I was a worrier, and that trait carried over into my adult life. Now I am beginning to understand Jesus' words in Matthew 6:25, 27 (NIV): *Therefore I tell you, do not worry about your life...Can any one of you by worrying add a single hour to your life?*

When I was a child, we often camped at Lost Lake near Mt. Hood in Oregon. What a beautiful place! To get to the campsite, we traveled narrow, windy mountain roads with steep drop offs at the side of the road. If another car came toward us going the other way, there was little room to pass. I used to worry about going over the edge. I think this was where my worrywart tendency was displayed and noticed by my family.

It is behaviors like worry that the Lord can take and completely remove from your life, just as things are erased from a dry erase board. My daughter had a dry erase board when she was younger. She could draw something and then wipe the board clean. We make mistakes and poor choices on the dry erase board of our life; when we seek the Lord's forgiveness, He takes the board and wipes it clean. Have you ever experienced this before? I have, time after time. He loves us enough to wash us clean. The Lord loves it when we come to Him in our pain. He delights in us. When we experience the cleansing of the Holy Spirit and our slate is white as snow, we are released into a freedom that we have never known. 2 Corinthians 3:16-18 (NIV) describes what it is like when the Lord cleanses us:

But whenever anyone turns to the Lord, the veil is taken away. Now the Lord is the Spirit, and where the Spirit of the Lord is, there is freedom. And we all, who with unveiled faces contemplate the Lord's glory, are being transformed into his image with ever-increasing glory, which comes from the Lord, who is the Spirit.

He takes the veil away! What a powerful statement! He wants to transform us; our responsibility is to turn to Him so He can do His work in us. As we all know, life is full of roadblocks and mess-ups, but I can tell you that every step of the way God is close by. He has His eraser ready. He does that for me and is waiting to do the same thing for you. Remember, becoming a Christian doesn't mean you don't have issues or recurring problems, but it does mean that you now have a direct line to Him through the Holy Spirit who lives in you.

Are you familiar with the story of Jesus' encounter with the woman caught in adultery (John 8)? What a powerful example of what Christ can do for us. The woman's accusers, wanting to trap Jesus into violating the Laws of Moses and stone the woman for her crime of adultery, made her stand before Jesus and the crowd.

But Jesus bent down and started to write on the ground with his finger. When they kept on questioning him, he straightened up and said to them, "Let any one of you who is without sin be the first to throw a stone at her." Again he stooped down and wrote on the ground.

*At this, those who heard began to go away one at a time, the
older ones first, until only Jesus was left, with the woman
still standing there. Jesus straightened up and asked her,
"Woman, where are they? Has no one condemned you?"*

*"No one, sir," she said.
"Then neither do I condemn you," Jesus declared.
"Go now and leave your life of sin."*

JOHN 8:6-11 (NIV)

What a gracious God we have! He stood before community leaders with this woman, defended her, wiped her slate clean, and removed her veil.

Now guys, let's get honest. Is there something in your life that you need to bring into the open? Is it the Internet, affairs, lust? You can name just about anything here. What is it? I ask that you would come to know the God I know, the One who set me free, and the One who has not condemned me for my sins. He told the adulterous woman to go and leave her life of sin. Wow! Imagine what your life will be like when you have a personal relationship with Him.

I have read a lot of books and spent hundreds of hours in counseling and treatment programs. You name it and I have probably done it over the past fifteen years. Yes, there were good things that came from the court-ordered counseling and treatment, but I needed something else, something more. It was with Pure Desire, that I found what I needed. The Pure Desire men's groups and Dr. Ted Robert's book titled *Pure Desire* have been major tools in my recovery. I saw first-hand how God can take the worst possible sins and wash people totally clean. I felt comfortable in my group and was able to trust the guys who have been fighting battles similar to mine. I knew I had to be with men who had a fresh start in life and were walking with other wounded warriors. Starting over is never easy. By His grace, God has gone before us time and time again, each time we start over.

As I continue writing this book, it is challenging to believe that God has brought me so far in what seems such a short time. Starting over with a clean slate, a new life! That is exactly what happens when we decide to live authentically and let God take control of our lives. He wants us to wholly submit to Him.

Can you look at your life and say you have given everything to God? I can't! I have a tendency to go to the altar and lay it all down, but as soon as I walk away, I grab a little piece to hang on to. So with that said, can we truly experience the cleansing that He has for us? This is something I struggle with at times with different issues. I know that He has cleansed me time and time again, and I long for the day when I can learn how to trust His every action in my life. However, I know there are still times my own insecurities block the cleansing of the Holy Spirit.

Recently I had a job change. Unhappy with the position I had, I actively looked for another opportunity. Finally, I found one and applied for a new job. After the first interview, I was asked to return to meet the top dog. After the second interview I was offered the job on the spot. As I was completing the paperwork, I came to the one question that I knew was coming; I stopped and prayed. I talked with the company managers about my felony conviction without going into detail. I took this opportunity to stand on God's Word that He was going to provide for me regardless of my past. They said they really appreciated my honesty and they still thought this was a good fit, so they hired me. This was the first time in an interview that I felt good about sharing my past. The Lord went before me and paved the way for me to get the job.

Everyone has different slates—different lives, different pasts—and they are all a mess. That is simply called being human. We each have our own issues that we can choose to bring to the forefront or stuff inside. However, when we stuff it inside and try to hide it, sooner or later those issues will always make their way to the surface.

I truly believe that for us to have our slates wiped clean and experience tremendous personal growth, we must go to God with everything. Set it all at the altar and don't take any pieces back. We live in a world where Satan will continue to attack us in every way possible. While the Lord loves to wash us clean, the enemy is always lurking around to muddy the waters. If we lose sight of who we are in Christ for one second, our thoughts get cloudy or we develop a sour heart, the enemy will unleash his attack on us. It is these very attacks that can make or break us. We ultimately have a choice to make.

The right thing to do is usually the hard thing to do. Making the right decisions becomes the toughest battles of our lives. One addiction or poor choice leads to another, and another, unless we continually go to the cross and lay it all down, asking God for forgiveness.

Let the Lord be the driver in your life and lead the way. I love Psalm 23. My prayer is that we all can learn to live out our lives and trust His paths for us.

The LORD is my shepherd, I lack nothing. He makes me lie down in green pastures, he leads me beside quiet waters, he refreshes my soul. He guides me along the right paths for his name's sake. Even though I walk through the darkest valley, I will fear no evil, for you are with me; your rod and your staff, they comfort me.

You prepare a table before me in the presence of my enemies. You anoint my head with oil; my cup overflows. Surely your goodness and love will follow me all the days of my life, and I will dwell in the house of the LORD forever.

PSALM 23 (NIV)

"Even though I walk through the valley" hits home with me. I cannot begin to count how many times I entered a valley, feeling alone. This Psalm gives me hope for the present and for things to come, knowing that He—my Lord and Savior—will be there.

CHAPTER 8

WALKING WITH GOD

Have you ever felt like you were on a leash and that the enemy was dangling a carrot in front of you? I have. At these times, we often forget or just don't think about from where we have come and Who brought us to this point. So many times in my life I have tried to get the carrot. Funny thing about the carrot: The enemy dangles it in front of us to divert our attention from Jesus. Your carrot may be sex, drugs, money, or other things. And we all have issues; we all have carrots. It's the "I want it now" syndrome. We are in such a hurry to fill the voids in our life that we don't stop to think about the consequences. That is when we find ourselves in trouble. Only one Person I know offers a hand every time. The love He has for us in our darkest hour is more than most of us can fathom.

You may be familiar with the poem *Footprints in The Sand*.[10] What a great description of our walk with Christ. At times when we don't think He is around, we come to realize later, it was at those times He was working behind the scenes on our behalf. God has come through so many times in my life, when I thought He was distant or didn't care. I was so out of control, I was surprised anyone wanted to be around me. God was so faithful and brought a blessing into my life following many of those desperate times. A great example was my criminal conviction; I truly thought that was the end of life for me. I look back now and see His footprints on the path carved out for me, His scars and the blood He shed for me. Scars in His hands from continuing to pull me out of the darkest pits in which I hid. And you know the great thing? Those scars are for all of us. Jesus died on the cross so we could be free.

Yet, in spite of everything He did for us that day, at times, we have chosen not to reach out to Him. Deuteronomy 30:15-16 (NIV) gives us a powerful look at what God asks of us:

See, I set before you today life and prosperity, death and destruction. For I command you today to love the Lord your God, to walk in obedience to him, and to keep his commands, decrees and laws; then you will live and increase, and the Lord your God will bless you in the land you are entering to possess.

What this passage does not say is that life is going to be easy. So many of us think that when we accept Christ in our lives God does the rest. I have been a believer almost my entire life and I still chose to walk away from Him. I chose to do things my way, on my own, regardless of the instructions and warnings in Scripture. God gives us opportunities to choose true life.

This day I call the heavens and the earth as witnesses against you that I have set before you life and death, blessings and curses. Now choose life, so that you and your children may live and that you may love the LORD your God, listen to his voice, and hold fast to him. For the LORD is your life, and he will give you many years in the land…

DEUTERONOMY 30:19-20 (NIV)

The Lord will carry us when we cannot carry ourselves. *He tends his flock like a shepherd; He gathers the lambs in his arms and carries them close to his heart; he gently leads those that have young* (Isaiah 40:11 NIV). For as much as God has carried me, I would love to see His chiropractor bill!

During my walk with God, I have asked Him numerous times, "Why, Lord? Why did you let this happen to me?" Funny thing is, His answers don't come when we want, and when He shows up, sometimes it's not fun. For every bad thing I did in my life, He showed me the way, He reached down and pulled me out of the pit and showered me with blessing after blessing, even though I felt undeserving. I was a lost soul and assumed He did not want anything to do with me, yet, He has been my number one running mate. He continues to lead me on new adventures daily, some easy and some painful. He continues to use my imperfections as a tool for me to seek a more intimate relationship with Him. Uncomfortable as I may be sometimes, He is leading, sculpting me into a new man. My walk with the Lord has been mostly one-sided. I would stray and take wrong turns and He would always redirect me, pushing or pulling me into a situation He knew I needed to experience. Isaiah 40:28-31 is a beautiful picture of His love and how He never gets tired of caring for me.

Do you not know? Have you not heard? The Lord is the ever-lasting God, the Creator of the ends of the earth. He will not grow tired or weary, and his understanding no one can fathom.
He gives strength to the weary and increases the power of the weak. Even youths grow tired and weary, and young men stumble and fall; but those who hope in the Lord will renew

*their strength. They will soar on wings like eagles; they will
run and not grow weary, they will walk and not be faint.*

ISAIAH 40:28-31 (NIV)

At the time I was convicted, God carried me into the courtroom,
He carried me out, He carried me through ten years of probation, and He continues to carry me today. No matter what we do
or where we go, good or bad, He is always there with His arms
extended just waiting for us to fall into His reach.

I can honestly say the safest place I've ever been is in the arms
of God; He must have thrown on hip waders and without hesi-
tation carried me through my junk. What the enemy meant for
destruction God uses to make us victorious. If we learn to walk
with Him, and be who He has called us to be, nothing can come
between God and us.

Trials and pain are like mysterious strangers who constantly
show up uninvited, walking hand-in-hand. Usually, when you
encounter one, the other is not far behind. No one can escape
their presence for long, for they are a common denominator
that unites us all. In my opinion, the greater a person's pain, the
greater potential they have to be a source of encouragement to
those around them who are also hurting and in need. After all,
how can one truly offer comfort if they themselves have never
been injured in some way? How can one provide emotional or
spiritual oxygen if they themselves have never known what it's
like to drown in sorrow?

Because of a personal relationship with Christ, joy can be our
constant companion. Since we know nothing comes into our
lives without purpose, when we face trials, we should be able to

feel a joyful anticipation for the resulting transformation. This does not mean that you should be excited about the pain you are experiencing, but there should be some anticipation for the work God is doing within you. We must have the mindset to persevere through the trials and be sharpened by them, so that we may be ready for the missions God gives us.

In a larger sense, however, the joy we feel is simply a byproduct of the One we know. During our trials, He is always there. He guides, protects, helps, and heals, so we are made more complete. James speaks about our desired attitude and approach to troubles:

> *Consider it pure joy, my brothers and sisters, whenever you face trials of many kinds, because you know that the testing of your faith develops perseverance. Let perseverance finish its work so that you may be mature and complete, not lacking anything.*
> JAMES 1:2-4 (NIV)

To be honest, there are moments when something within me still rails against being joyful in times of pain and trials. Like when someone cuts me off in traffic or when I have to deal with the difficulties of life. Am I really supposed to count that all joy? And what about when I'm faced with a bigger problem? What then? God promises never to leave or forsake us, but He never promises that this life would be a cakewalk. As a matter of fact, His Son forewarned us that it would be otherwise.

> *"I have told you these things, so that in me you may have peace. In this world you will have trouble. But take heart! I have overcome the world."*
> JOHN 16:33 (NIV)

It is easier to persevere when we also consider God's promise of 1 Corinthians 10:13 (NIV):

No temptation has overtaken you except what is common to mankind. And God is faithful; he will not let you be tempted beyond what you can bear. But when you are tempted, he will also provide a way out so that you can endure it.

We, in and of ourselves, are not strong enough; but while we are walking with God we will be given the strength to bear any burden and be provided a way through any situation we encounter. The "way out" for you and me could mean counseling and/or a men's purity group. So take heart! Walk boldly and without fear through any trials, knowing that the One who created everything is walking hand-in-hand with you.

ASK YOURSELF…

Am I able to look for God's hand in my trials or am I focused either on the pain or the solution? Do I let worry overtake me?

PRAY…

God, help me see Your plan in my pain. I want to walk with Your joy so that my trials may serve Your purpose. Provide me with Your strength to persevere on the journey to a healthy lifestyle.

TAKE ACTION…

Take five minutes to make some notes about where you've been in regard to your pain and past choices, where you are now, and where you would like God to take you in the future. How have you changed or grown as a result of reading this book or beginning to be honest about your situation?

CHAPTER 9

GOD'S CALL

Have you identified your God-given call? When I finally figured out that I had a God-given call, I had many steps to take before I began. Many of those I shared in previous chapters. God can place a call on your life, but He won't set it in motion until He knows you are ready. No matter what type of call we experience, each of us must first begin to face our pain, for it is when we are broken that Christ will begin to fine-tune us. The fine-tuning is not always an easy process. Pain, Anger, Frustration! Yes, we experience it all in our times of growth. His call on our lives is just that, His call. Not ours, but His. And, when we truly hear from God, we need to get ready for a wild ride.

Nothing is easy when it comes to Christian living. Things actually seem harder at times, and they are. We become the target when we make the choice to walk with God. In reality, as a Christian we are always the target, but when we are living the way of the world we don't realize what we are doing. We fill the voids in our lives with "stuff" and society preaches that the more possessions we have, the more successful we will be and the more friends we will have.

When I truly understood God's call on my life, my choice was obvious. I chose to pour into guys struggling with sexual addiction. My choice to listen to God allowed the Holy Spirit to begin to change my heart. For more than ten years of doing Pure Desire men's groups, I have been blessed by the stories that other men share. It is often during those times of sharing their painful stories that the Holy Spirit will enter and become an overpowering Presence. I always tell the guys that when someone in the group is in crisis, we are there for that individual. When a man shares his pain, the door opens for others to experience healing, revealing something within them that has not yet been addressed. Tremendous things happen in our men's groups during times of Holy Spirit ministering; marriages healed, families healed, and lives forever changed.

I love the fact that I can go to my Pure Desire group and not be afraid to share about my life and myself. These groups have played a significant and essential part of many men's paths to healing. When I heard God call me to be there for guys who are struggling, I could not turn my back. I am so thankful for the men who didn't turn their backs on me when I first came to a group.

We all have a calling and purpose in life. Just as God called Moses to lead the Israelites out of captivity, so He calls each of us for His purpose: *But I have raised you up for this very purpose, that I might show you my power and that my name might be proclaimed in all the earth* (Exodus 9:16 NIV).

And we know that in all things God works for the good of those who love him, who have been called according to his purpose (Romans 8:28 NIV). What great words for us to hold onto! The Lord has called us and has a purpose for us. I believe with all my heart that God's call for me and my life will be more fulfilling than any call I could ever place on myself. In the 1500s, Martin Luther spoke these words that continue to ring true today for those who seek God:

All who call on God in true faith, earnestly from the heart, will certainly be heard, and will receive what they have asked and desired, although not in the hour or in the measure of the very thing they ask. Yet they will obtain something greater and more glorious than they had dared to ask.[11]

ALL who call on God. Not Him calling on us, because He has been calling on us for a long time; we just refused to listen. But the moment we truly call on Him is when we can begin to see Him and His work in our lives clearly. I have really good days and really bad days, but I know that God's hand is on my life and that He has called me to be a warrior! A fighter for men.

I like the words of Coach Eddie Robinson: *Leadership, like coaching is fighting for the hearts and souls of men, and getting them to believe in you.*[12] We have the greatest leader of all time; He is fighting for us. He has been molding us from before we were born; he has been coaching us, carrying us through tough times, and yet there are so many of us who do not believe in Him. Nonetheless, He still has His arms open to us, waiting for us to give it all to Him. You will never understand your God-given purpose if you do not fully unload all your fears and worries on God. When He calls us we must choose to respond, and place our life in His hands.

Do you have a relationship with Jesus Christ? If you don't, it is really easy to ask Him into your life. You can ask God right now to fill that empty place in your life and reveal His love and calling for you. I would like to pray the sinner's pray with you now. This must come from your heart. I hope this will help you to invite Jesus into your heart and life. This prayer is here only as a guide; please feel free to pour out your heart to Jesus in your own words.

Heavenly Father, have mercy on me, a sinner. I believe in You and that Your word is true. I believe that Jesus Christ is the Son of the Living God and that He died on the cross so that I may now have forgiveness for my sins and eternal life. I know that without You in my heart my life is meaningless.

I believe that you, Father God, raised Him from the dead. Please, Jesus, forgive me for every sin I have ever committed or done in my heart. Please, Lord Jesus, forgive me and come into my heart as my personal Lord and Savior today. I need you to be my God and my Friend. I give You my life and ask You to take full control from this moment on; I pray this in the name of Jesus Christ. Amen.

Martin Luther also said, "*I have held many things in my hands, and I have lost them all; but whatever I have placed in God's hands, that I still posses.*"[13] Seems so simple a task, yet we all have a hard time doing it. We bring something to the altar to let it go. When we turn around to walk away, we reach back and take hold of it once again. I still struggle with fully letting go. All I know is that God gave me third and fourth and fifth chances at life—probably more chances than that. Dr. Ted Roberts once told me that he had never seen someone experience such blessing in the midst of doing the wrong thing. That is what God has done in my life, and He can do it for you. Now when blessings come my way, I see them in a much healthier light. I am able to see that my value does not come from what I want for my life, but from what God has planned for my life.

Guys, we are all called to be fighters. Warriors for Christ. To go out and fight for those men struggling with sexual addiction who cannot fight for themselves right now. Our battle is best fought when we band together in an accountability group, such as a Pure Desire men's group. I truly believe there is no greater call than to serve the Lord and be on the front lines of the battlefield. We live in a world today that is setup to destroy us. The life God has for us in these rough times can be amazing when we open up our hearts and let God lead us into battle. The battle has already been won; Jesus fought it for us when He died on the cross. Our job is to take action when He calls upon us. I never want to forget that. I simply pray I can be half the man as some of the men who have stood with me during the battle of my healing journey.

CHAPTER 10

THE VICTORY

When I started to think about writing this book, I found myself feeling great fear. Guys, I wrote this book for you. As I look back over the months of writing, I realize just how far I have come. I have relived some terrible times, examined the things I did, and remembered the people I hurt—which caused me to experience pain I thought I would never feel this side of my addiction. I thank the Lord every day that He has brought me to the point where I can share with you words of hope and encouragement. This took a lot of courage to write. I was forced to be honest with myself and look at my past in a new light. My past is just that, my past. I now have the joy of knowing that Christ is with me now and in the future.

But those who hope in the LORD will renew their strength.
They will soar on wings like eagles;
they will run and not grow weary,
they will walk and not be faint.

ISAIAH 40:31 (NIV)

Guys, put your name in that scripture: *I,* _____ , *who hope in the Lord will renew my strength. I will soar on wings like eagles; I will run and not grow weary, I will walk and not be faint.* Pretty powerful when you read it like that!

My prayer is that, as you have walked through this book with me, I have given you a sense of hope. I know, first hand, how tough it is. This battle we have faced all our lives is one we cannot win alone. When I made the choice to become brutally honest, I felt the Holy Spirit touch my life. In our Pure Desire men's group we always talk about *vulnerable transparency*. It's just what it sounds like—you get to the point where you make the choice not to hide anymore and make the choice to let God take over in your life. When you reach this point, you allow the Holy Spirit to begin to do miraculous things in your life.

Finally, brothers and sisters, rejoice! Strive for full restoration, encourage one another, be of one mind, live in peace. And the God of love and peace will be with you.
2 CORINTHIANS 13:11 (NIV)

We are called to love our brothers. We are called to show them mercy and grace, and encourage them in their times of struggle. What does your victory dance look like? I hope you experience it soon.

Looking back over my life, I see many small victories. If you have hung in there with me through this book and are currently struggling, there is help. Guys, I know it's scary and shameful. I know what you're experiencing. If you are saying, "If he really knew me, if he really knew my struggle…" But I do know! This may be the one decision you make in your life that will have eternal rewards. We don't have to life a life of shame or guilt anymore. We can truly be set free.

A few years ago, I got a letter from a gentleman in prison. He was going to be incarcerated for many, many years. He wrote about how he had struggled with sexual addiction his entire life and that it cost him his freedom. I remember sharing with him that he had a choice to make regardless of his situation and where he would be living for many years. I told him he may never see freedom outside the prison walls again, but that he could experience Freedom in Christ. To be honest with you, guys, when we are living our secret lives we are holding ourselves in prison, right in the open, where everyone can see us. If that is you, can you imagine your life completely free from what you are going through right now? Imagine what life would be like without all the baggage you are trying to hide. You can experience life the way God intended.

The victory is truly ours. Jesus fought our battle for us so that we can live in Him. Even though He has gone before us and fought the battle, we still must choose God. Are you ready to make that choice? As you read the sinner's prayer in the last chapter, I hope that it began to spark something in you. The toughest thing for a man to do is to admit he has failed. We have to lay down our pride and accept the fact we have sinned and that our sin has created pain for others. We have to come to the realization that the only way we can experience the true victory, is to let the Lord work in our lives. Go back and re-read the prayer in the last chapter and open your heart to what the Lord can do in you and for you.

When I went to my first Pure Desire men's group, I was scared because I did not know how the guys would react to my story. But they spoke words of encouragement, hope, and peace over me. (Thank you, Mike!) It only took one guy in that group to show me that I was worth the fight, I was important to God and

I mattered, even when I felt like I didn't. I knew I could count on him to listen to what I was going through; I respected him enough to allow him to speak into my life. These are the type of guys we need in our lives—men with whom we can be vulnerably transparent. So many of us have issues with trusting people because we, too, have been betrayed. We can learn to trust God and others, and when we do, we will begin to walk in victory.

Those who know your name trust in you,
for you, LORD, have never forsaken those who seek you.
PSALM 9:10 (NIV)

Trust. Sounds easy, and to some extent it is. It's easy to say we trust the Lord, but we have to connect our words with our hearts and invite Him in. Scripture says He will never forsake those who seek Him. If you have not done so already, I encourage you to seek Him. Take those first steps toward freedom. If you have not heard Jason Upton's version of the song *Freedom Reigns in This Place*, please listen to it. The song is a great picture of God's freedom that began for me right where I was standing at the time I looked to Him and invited Him into my life. I know what Christ did for me and I know He will do the same for you.

If sharing my story has helped you in anyway, praise God. Without Him, my words are nothing. Knowing that I can walk in victory did not make this any easier to write; in fact, this is one of the hardest things I've done in my life. But the fact I am sharing with you tells me that this just the beginning of what God has for me. Many men out there are destroying what God wants for them. I pray that all of you would see the truth that He does love you, has a call on your life, and calls you to live in victory. All our stories are different, yet the same. We all have fallen short of the

Glory of God, still He calls each and every one of us to Himself and to be victorious in battle.

> *But you give us victory over our enemies,*
> *you put our adversaries to shame.*
> PSALM 44:7 (NIV)

> *With God we will gain victory,*
> *and he will trample down our enemies.*
> PSALM 60:12 (NIV)

What's next for you? If you are walking a path similar to my old path, please get help. I know you can do it. I will pray that you find the way—God's Way. God gives us freewill to make our own decisions. You only have two choices: change or not change. I pray you will choose God and allow Christ to change your life.

I hope and pray that as you have read my story you are inspired. I know you can overcome the battles you are facing. Remember that the Lord is preparing a victory celebration for you.

Lord, I pray Your peace for each man who reads this book. Give each one courage to choose You. May this story help others be encouraged and hopeful for personal and family healing. Let each and every man who struggles the way I did realize they are not alone. I pray for other Kingdom warriors to surround each wounded warrior on their healing journey. God, may each man begin to trust You and believe that You are walking with them. Amen.

CHAPTER 11

A FRESH START

Starting over, making a fresh start is what most of us think about at the beginning of a new year. We start off a new year with the resolve to make changes, but as the months go by, the passion we had when we decided to make the change fizzles away. Starting over and changing old behaviors is hard. This story is about making those changes, being committed to the process, and having people in your life who will keep you on track.

A person who struggles with addiction has a battle that is so deep in the brain that it makes them feel powerless to change. They want to stop, and try to stop many times. But they fail every time. They want to change. They want to start over. But how? Why is it so hard?

After struggling over twenty-five years with sexual addiction and the coping behaviors I had put in place, I began to think that things would never change. But deep within me, something was stirring. God was relentless in His pursuit of me, constantly letting me know how much He loved me and that I was worth changing. Even to this day He continues to mold me and prune those areas in my life that need to die.

The turning point for me was facing my addiction head on. As you may recall, my story includes abuse and addiction and how it affected my family and friends. I had to begin to get brutally honest about what I was doing. When I faced losing my family and faced many years in prison, God had my full attention. Honestly facing what I had done started me on the healthier path I am on now. I was given a second chance. God has some great plans for me. My responsibility was to make the decision to be obedient and start fully trusting God, which is something I had never completely done before.

Starting in 1997, when I got help with my sexual addiction, I thought that was the only thing I needed to work on. Oh, how wrong I was! Part of changing and starting fresh is growth. Along with growth comes pain. Well, yes, there was more pain to come. God started revealing my issues with money, lying, stealing, you name it. I thought this would all be taken care of when I started dealing with the sexual part—not so! The term "comorbidity" applies when someone has multiple addictions; one addiction may seem to be under control, but the same addictive patterns bring other addictive behaviors to the forefront. As I worked on my sexual addiction, my other addictive behaviors surfaced more strongly. Lying was an obvious addiction for me. I would say or do anything to cover up a problem. I stole money and items because I told myself I deserved it. Now, I am thankful that those other addictive behaviors surfaced, so I could also work on them. I learned that God will first teach us a lesson and then show Himself to us in the midst of our poor decisions.

You may remember Paul Harvey and his iconic *The Rest of The Story*. What you are reading right now is my *Rest of the Story*. In

June 2015, I was working a good job that paid well and had been promoted to management. I was offered a full time position at Pure Desire Ministries. After being in Pure Desire groups for almost eighteen years, and being a leader for most of those years, I reached a time in my life that required me to step out in faith and take on a new challenge for Pure Desire. You would think that doing what I was doing for so long would make a new step easy, but it was a difficult decision. After much prayer, I took the job. Now I get to share my story on a daily basis with men all over the world, and I get to walk with men as they begin the process of becoming free. What better job could you have than to provide support and encourage for men and their families?

Dr. Ted Roberts, co-founder of Pure Desire Ministries, says that we are wounded in community and we are healed in community. To learn this truth in new ways, I have recently stepped back into serving in my church, after having stepped away from active ministry there due to being wounded by leadership seven years ago. After talking with the some of the staff at the church and the staff at Pure Desire, it seemed wise for me to take that next step. I truly believe that this is the time God has set aside for me to pursue church ministry. And, through this next season of my life, especially at church, there is healing taking place. A fresh start!

I had to examine what was holding me back from stepping once again into leadership at the church. I ended up looking at the situation like an injury. I grew up playing many sports, and along with sports came injuries. Broken bones, cuts, bruises, knee surgery, you name it. My mom once said that between my brother and me, our medical bills built part of the local hospital. While growing up, every season, we were at the hospital for something.

So I had to look at re-entering leadership like those injuries. We all need rehabilitation in some area. We enter rehab to help recover and regain strength from our injuries just as we must do rehab to strengthen our hearts and our minds from mental and emotional wounds.

God calls every one of us in our brokenness to a fresh start—a start that God knows we can handle, a start that requires each of us to step out of our comfort zone. And, until we are ready to step out, He continues to work on our hearts. As I look back over the last eighteen years, I have been in some intense rehab. Pure Desire helped save my life, and has helped restore my faith in people, including those closest to me.

Many of us just want to start over and leave all the junk behind. But what we fail to realize is that the junk we thought we left behind is still attached to us. It is sitting in the passenger seat right beside you on the way to work in the morning, sitting on your desk like a paper weight, ready for you to pick up and run with all over again. When you are faced with life's most crucial decisions, which way are you going to go? Who are you going to turn to? You choose—the old you and your old behaviors, or the new you, the changed you.

There is always a kind of awkward phase when we finally reach a point of health. The tipping point so to speak. You are almost to the point where you can finally let go of everything, yet you are unable. Why? God has brought you to this point. He has pulled you out of the pit of hell. Why can't you fully TRUST Him? What does it look like? There were periods during my healing, when I trusted no one, including God. To be honest, I still have a hard time trusting Him with everything, but I am working on it.

So many of us stop moving forward and become stagnant after a victory, especially when it involves a long and hard battle. It is at that very point when once again you are faced with tough decisions. Do you tell yourself you are done and can move on? At that point, I believe one of the only options is to devote yourself to helping others and to give back to others what was given to you. In some ways, this was an easy choice for me. Why wouldn't I give back to a ministry that saved my life? I would be dead or in prison if it were not for God and Pure Desire. God is using my junk as a tool for me to help others.

We all have life experiences that have helped mold us into who we are. I am not proud of my addictions and how they impacted others, but I am proud of who I am becoming. I have been blessed with some great opportunities over the past few years, including helping to run a small family-owned business with my brother and sister-in-law. That alone is a true miracle. The relationship I now have with my brother and his family is great! Even my relationship with my niece has been fully restored. We are closer today than I ever thought possible. It is something that I never imagined would happen. God has great plans for us.

It is important to remember that the healing process takes work and we have to put forth the effort. Steps need to be taken, and if you are committed to the process, you will see great results in every aspect of your life. For me, making the right decisions during my healing process has led me to better job opportunities. Every step of the way, each job became better because I was at a place in my life where I trusted God for what I needed. He blessed me every step of the way.

What does your story look like? I encourage you to write out your story. Share your current situation and reality, what God has done in your life or what you want Him to do, and any miracles you have experienced or want to experience. Remember, there is tremendous power in your story. During your healing journey, sharing your story may be the one thing that helps save a life (maybe your own!), a marriage, or even a child. We never know when God will use us, but He will use you and your story.

I hope more than anything that I have encouraged you to never give up. Fight the good fight. Are you ready to partner with other men and fight the battle with them, and help them write their story as you write yours? It is time to stand together arm-in-arm with your brothers and stop fighting alone.

As I enter a new season in my life, I am in the midst of another battle. I am totally all-in for Christ. Yet with all the clarity and focus I have, I still do not know what this season will look like or the challenges and battles ahead. God knows, and He knows my heart's desire and my struggles. He is stretching and molding me for the purpose for which He created me. It requires me to be flexible, and requires a 100% trust in Him. I am ready for this. I am ready to stomp on hell and take back what the enemy has taken away.

God has taken my pain and turned it into a new career for me—a blessing I never saw coming. A blessing and a call I take on whole-heartedly. I owe so much to the staff of Pure Desire and the men and women who have been in my corner for so many years. God knew what I needed; He put the circumstances in place and allowed me to make the choice to work for Pure Desire or walk away. Making the right decisions come with growing pains and tough lessons. But I believe the best is yet to come. God has healed me on the inside and continues to be my strength and security. He chose me, and for that I am thankful.

"Nevertheless, I will bring health and healing to it; I will heal my people and will let them enjoy abundant peace and security."
JEREMIAH 33:6 (NIV)

Note: Throughout this book I have mentioned Pure Desire groups and other resources that been valuable and useful in my recovery. Look in the **Resources** *section at the back of this book for more information.*

RESOURCES

Pure Desire | Gresham, Oregon
puredesire.org | 503-489-0230

Pure Desire Ministries has practical answers that deal not only with the struggle of sexual and other addictions, but also with the family systems that fuel the issues.

Resources available at puredesire.org/store include:

- *Conquer Series: The Battle Plan for Purity.* A DVD series hosted by Dr. Ted Roberts. Study guide available. (Produced by Jeremy & Tiana Wiles, KingdomWorks Studios.)

- *Seven Pillars of Freedom Men's Workbook, Journal,* and *Leader's Guide* by Dr. Ted Roberts

- *Top Gun: Flight Manual for Young Men in a Pornified World* by Dr. Ted Roberts & Bryan Roberts

- *Betrayal & Beyond: Fashioning a Courageous Heart* (for women who have been betrayed) by Diane Roberts

- *Eight Pillars to Freedom* (for women with love and/or sex addiction) by Diane Roberts

- *Behind the Mask: Authentic Living for Young Women* by Rebecca Bradley & Diane Roberts

- *Hope for Men: Healing for Broken Trust* (for men who have been betrayed) by Dr. Ted & Diane Roberts

- *Pure Desire* by Dr. Ted Roberts

ENDNOTES

1. Eddie Robinson, College Football Coach. 1919-2007. http://sports.espn.go.com/ncf/news/story?id=2825256

2. Vince Lombardi, Pro Football Coach. www.brainyquote.com/quotes/quotes/v/vincelomba151240.html

3. Ted Roberts, *Pure Desire* (Ventura, CA: Regal Books, 2008)

4. Civil War Trust: Saving America's Civil War Battlefields. http://www.civilwar.org/education/history/faq/

5. Jacquelyn Ekern, MS, LPC. http://www.addictionhope.com/sexual-addiction

6. Timothy Light. http://www.helium.com/items/1809919-anger-feelings-mad-mind-body-soul-pain-numb-actions-angry

7. Diane Roberts, *Betrayal & Beyond Workbook III*. (Gresham, OR: Pure Desire Ministries International, 2010) 94.

8. Corrie Ten Boom, *The Hiding Place* (Boston: G.K. Hall, 1973).

9. Stephen Covey, *The 7 Habits of Highly Effective People: Powerful Lessons in Personal Change*. (New York: Free Press, 2004).

10. Mary Stevenson. "Footprints in the Sand" http://www.footprints-inthe-sand.com

11. Martin Luther. http://thinkexist.com/quotation/all_who_call_on_god_in_true_faith-earnestly_from/164467.html

12. Eddie Robinson, College Football Coach. http://www.inspirational-quotes-and-quotations.com/coaching-quotes.html

13. Martin Luther. http://thinkexist.com/quotation/i_have_held_many_things_in_my_hands-and_i_have/169725.html